Brother to Brother

YOU DON'T HAVE TO DIE WITH PROSTATE CANCER

Thomas L. Walker

Survivor and Author

eternal gold
PUBLISHERS

Brother To Brother
You Don't Have To Die With Prostate Cancer

Copyright 1998 by Thomas L. Walker

Eternal Gold Publishers
P. O. Box 4633
Rocky Mount, NC 27803
(252) 443-5605

To reach us on the Internet: **www.egpub.com**
e-mail: **eternalgoldpub@bbnp.com**

ISBN 0-9665465-0-4

First Published in 1998

U.S. $15.95
Canada $17.95

Table of Contents

Dedication

This book is dedicated to my wife, Joyce, whom I have grown to recognize as my African Queen. Thanks, Joyce, for 35 years of dedication, love and support (31 years of marriage; 4 years of courtship). Thanks for sharing the journey with me from the initial visit to the urologist, when I learned that I had prostate cancer, to that glorious day in New Port Richey, Florida when Dr. Jerrold Sharkey, M.D., F.A.C.S., told us that they found no traces of cancer in my prostate. Please be assured that as long as God gives me health and strength, I'll be the wind beneath your wings.

Acknowledgments

Words are inadequate to express my sincere appreciation to the many friends and loved ones who contributed to the writing of this book.

Special thanks to my wife and children for the support base they provided during my experience with prostate cancer and their assistance in writing this book. To Teresa and her husband, Donnie, and to Tim and his wife, Annette, thanks for your support and assistance with proofreading. I shall always cherish the support shown by my mother and sister in my times of crises.

Special thanks to Ms. Debra Harding who served as typist, proofreader, and research assistant without which this project could not have been completed.

I am grateful to the members of my congregation who continuously besought God on my behalf for my healing. I am deeply indebted to Pastor Steve Lewis and the Englewood Baptist Church for the use of their facilities in completing this project.

I am especially grateful to the many physicians, whose expertise and skill contributed to my complete recovery: Joseph Whisnant, M.D., my local urologist; Jerrold Sharkey, M.D., F.A.C.S., at the Urology Health Center in New Port Richey, Florida; Samuel Wesonga, M.D., our family physician; and Frederick Ellwanger, M.D., Radiologist at Nash General Hospital. My dear friend, E. C. Land, M.D. of Greenville, North Carolina, deserves much praise for his encouragement as I developed this project.

Acknowledgments

Special thanks to Emerson Harrison, M.D., FACS, whom I've known from a child. Not only am I proud of his great accomplishments, but I appreciate the countless hours he spent reviewing this book to be sure the medical statistics were accurate. I am grateful to the other physicians who read and critiqued this book: E. C. Land, M.D.; Lisa Nelson-Robinson, M.D.; Jerrold Sharkey, M.D., F.A.C.S.; Stuart K. Todd, M.D.; Joseph D. Whisnant, Jr., M.D.; and Samuel Wesonga, M.D.

I am also thankful to Patrick Ellis and my sister, Retha Archer, who assisted in proofreading.

Special acknowledgment to Bob Samuels, Chairman of the National Prostate Cancer Coalition. I've never met a man so passionately involved with a mission. Clearly, Bob's mission is "ending prostate cancer as a serious health concern for men and their families."

Special thanks to Congresswoman Eva M. Clayton, who not only encouraged me during my hours of struggle, but inspired me through her untiring efforts to serve others.

No list of acknowledgments would be complete without my good friend Bro. Ernest Bulluck, who comforted me through my experience with prostate cancer after having similar experiences.

Legal Statement

While I am not a medical doctor, I am a survivor of one of the most serious diseases known to man, prostate cancer. Out of my own experiences and research, I am providing information that I trust will be helpful in saving many lives and answering many questions in the minds of the readers.

The information in this book is not meant to be a medical prescription. The author, publisher, and reviewing physicians have no liability or responsibility to any person or persons with respect to any harm, loss or damage caused or alleged to be caused directly or indirectly by the information contained in this book.

I am thoroughly convinced that all the information provided in this book is accurate in accordance with statistics from bonafide cancer agencies and associations. If there are any questions about any of the contents of this book, feel free to ask your physician or medical advisor.

Physician Reviews

The diagnosis of prostate cancer is a life changing event for any man with this problem. Reverend Walker has done an outstanding job in enumerating the emotional and physical problems of the disease. He has also taken you step-by-step through the process and diagnosis to getting various opinions on treatment alternatives to making the decision for his treatment. The major lesson of the book is what Reverend Walker speaks over and over and over again about—don't be ashamed to go get a checkup. . .

Jerrold Sharkey, M.D., FACS
New Port Richey, Florida

I have no doubt that this book will save men's lives. I appreciate his attention to the medical detail and the obvious time and diligence required for a layman to compile this excellent volume. I can only hope with Reverend Walker that more men, particularly African American men, will avail themselves of the information and insight in this book. . . *Jospeh D. Whisnant, Jr., M.D.*
Rocky Mount, North Carolina

Most often if I can get a lay person to communicate medical information it is received with more impact to my target audience. Your first-hand perspective adds additional potency and urgency to your message. Personally, I look forward to promoting your book in the Greenville area and only hope you will agree to the many opportunities to bring your message to our community which will come with the book's publication. . .

E. C. Land, M.D.
Greenville, North Carolina

I enjoyed reading your book. It is clearly written, extremely personal, and directly to the point. Prostate cancer, as well as breast, colon and lung, are prime killers in the African American community and our people need to take heed and <u>listen</u>! Your book is a perfect vehicle for this. . .
Lisa Nelson-Robinson, M.D.
Rocky Mount, North Carolina

I think your work is excellent and I enjoyed reading it personally. I was also struck by your devotion to your wife and also her chapter in the book.. .
Stuart K. Todd, M.D.
Rocky Mount, North Carolina

(See Appendix B for complete Physician Reviews)

Layman Reviews

Although I have a decade before I am chronologically inducted into the 40+ group, this book has made me more keenly aware of the effects of prostate cancer. This book is quite practical. Rev. Walker carefully outlines an aggressive action plan on the final pages of the book. If this plan is followed, we can soon eliminate prostate cancer.

James Earl Sledge

As the brother-in-law of the author, I've had few things to impact my life as has this book. Strangely enough, Rev. Walker and his wife visited our home in Richmond, Virginia only one day prior to submitting this book to the printer. Little did he know, I was scheduled to visit my urologist three days later about prostate concerns. When I read through the draft of the book, it completely enlightened me on how I should approach my physician and what I was to expect.

Clarence Archer

Dr. Walker's book is the Rosetta Stone for helping "brothers" avoid, confront and survive prostate cancer.

Eustace A. Dixon, Ph.D.

Dr. Walker's book sheds a tremendous amount of light on a health problem that knows no racial or cultural boundaries. All men are in dire need of the information and education this book has to offer. And while it focuses on prostate cancer, what it really does is challenge men to be and remain health conscious throughout their lives.

Jerry L. Harper

Foreword

Prostate cancer has significantly touched the lives of hundreds of thousands of men, particularly African American men. In the last five to seven years, interest and awareness have heightened in our communities. Unfortunately, prostate cancer continues to be the second leading cause of cancer deaths in men. African American men are particularly effected by this disease. The incidence rates are nearly two times higher for African American men than white men. The good news is that early detection and treatment increase the potential for cure.

The American Cancer Society and the American Foundation for Urologic Disease (A.F.U.D.) have sponsored programs that have increased awareness, promoted the importance of prostate health, and the value of early detection of prostate cancer.

This book is a must read for all men and family members of men who are age forty or older. **Brother To Brother** is an excellent synopsis and review of one prostate cancer survivor's experiences from beginning to cure. Dr. Walker has written an easy to understand, patient-friendly book that covers many of the common concerns of those afflicted with prostate cancer. Remember, the patient that is educated about prostate cancer, will experience less fear about diagnosis and treatment. This book is a valuable tool in educating patients about prostate cancer.

Emerson E. Harrison, M.D. FACS
Prostate Cancer Specialist/Urologist
Atlanta Urological Consultants, P.C. (Atlanta, Georgia)
Assistant Clinical Professor
Department of Surgery
Emory University School of Medicine

Preface

In recent years, prostate cancer has become an issue of public forums, talk shows, and the focus of media campaigns. Still, it has not received the level of research funding as some other cancers.

As I look around at men and notice what appears to be troubled minds, I often wonder if the reasons are health-related concerns. How many of their lives have been devastated by the knowledge that they have prostate cancer? How many of them are so immobilized by the news that they do not know which way to turn? How many of them refuse to do anything? How many of them have recognized that their inactivity has led them to a point of no return? How many of them are struggling to keep it from their friends, associates, and even family? More importantly, how many are struggling with pre-cancerous symptoms but refuse to seek medical attention?

These concerns have grown out of my own experience of being diagnosed with prostate cancer. In this book, you will see how God has led me through a process that resulted in my miraculous healing. I believe that every man who is stricken with this disease and who takes early proactive steps can experience the same healing.

Introduction

Like most of the American public, I had not given too much thought to prostate cancer. . . until it affected me. It is strange how one can have an experience that can force him to see life from a totally different perspective.

For years, I considered myself to be in relatively good health, although I had bouts with the black plague for African Americans--high blood pressure. I attributed this condition to the fast-paced life I had led for twenty-five years as Pastor of one of the largest churches in eastern North Carolina. Along with my pastorship came a ministry of music that I would try to keep afloat. I had recorded eight albums, some containing gospel music and some preaching. Although the majority of the proceeds from this ministry went toward the building of a new church, I worked to stay on top of it for personal reasons.

Every Fall, I would run myself nearly ragged as I traveled to and from churches throughout the United States and abroad conducting week-long revivals. For twelve years, I was known as a preacher who was also a politician. As I basked in the glory of being seen as one of the most powerful Black men in Eastern North Carolina, I gladly dealt with the physical exertion that came with that glory. Although my hectic schedule kept me in constant need of sleep, I looked great. At least everyone told me I did.

As my life progressed, I had every reason to be happy. My son had been called into the ministry and served as Pastor of his own church. My daughter had finished law school and had become an attorney. My ministry was growing, although not as fast as I wished. At age 47, I looked forward to a future of enjoying my wife Joyce, my three grandchildren, and continuing to brave the lifestyle to which I had become accustomed.

Aside from a neurological condition that Joyce (my wife of 31 years) endured, sickness had not reared its head in my immediate family. She is stricken with a rare degenerative disease called "oligopontocerrebullar atrophy," that affects her neurological functions. When she learned of my condition, she put all of her energies into encouraging me. Having no regard for her own health, it appeared that all of her concern, compassion, and love was turned toward me.

As I was dealing with the agonizing reality that sickness had stricken my body, I promised God that if He healed me, I would not only glorify Him forever and ever, but I would attempt to write a book about my experience with prostate cancer. After handling the anxiety that came with choosing a treatment that was right for me, and all of the issues that I had to resolve within myself during the process, I now find much joy in sharing my miraculous story of healing and deliverance with others.

Chapter 1

From One Brother to Another

Am I my brother's keeper?
Genesis 4:9

Most of us are familiar with an episode in the first book of the Bible concerning two brothers Cain and Abel. You recall Cain killed his brother Abel in a jealous rage. The question was then raised by God to Cain, "Where is thy brother?" Cain responded by asking God a question. "Am I my brother's keeper?" This question has been raised by many generations in an attempt to justify indifference, insensitivity, and irresponsibility. However, I declare today that although I may not be my brother's keeper, I am clearly my brother's brother. So from one brother to another, please read on and live.

My brother, please allow me to be very transparent, and yet, not preach to you. We, men, for the most part, are very private and unemotional--even about our own health and well-being. However, pride will only get us an early grave. I cannot overemphasize the importance of you becoming as knowledgeable as possible about your own health, especially the health of your prostate.

Unfortunately, many of us have for too long regulated our health by street conversations, barber shop gossip, and buddy-to-buddy myths. Many men think a visit to the urologist will ultimately endanger their manhood and render them sexually impotent, especially if the doctor starts "messing around" with his prostate. From a personal experience, I plead with you to find a good urologist and set up an annual appointment to have your prostate thoroughly examined. Statistics suggest that this is extremely important for men 40 and above. That is why I am convinced that all men over 40 should have an annual prostate exam and PSA (prostate specific antigen) test.

Who Is This Book Written For?

Men of all ages and ethnic backgrounds, family members, wives, friends, or anyone whose life is touched by an adult male need to read this book. This book has a serious message for every man who is over 40 years of age. This issue of prostate disease will likely touch your life (if you're a man) or the life of a male relative or acquaintance at some point. I strongly encourage all men, especially African American men, to read this book with a sense of urgency. Statistics show that African American men are two times more likely to have prostate cancer than other ethnic groups. According to Don Speaks, Conference Coordinator for "Brothers Can We Talk About It?," a conference held in Atlanta, Georgia on May 2, 1998, ". . if black people, especially black men do not start taking control of our personal health status we will be on the verge of extinction by the end of the 21st century!" I agree with Mr. Speaks' statement.

Why I Wrote This Book

One might ask why I would engage in the time and discipline necessary to compile all the information contained in this book. After all, my schedule is overwhelming, as it is. Consider pastoring over 1,200 parishioners, preparing teaching and preaching materials for a minimum of four worship services and Bible studies per week, in addition to counseling, hospital visitations and all the other unexpected interruptions such as deaths and tragedies that inevitably confront my parishioners. In the book of all books (The Holy Bible), Hosea 4:6 says, "My people are destroyed for lack of knowledge. . ." I've always heard the cliché, "what you don't know won't hurt you." Prostate cancer begs to differ. The more you know about prostate cancer, the better your chances of survival.

I will always appreciate my doctor, Dr. Joseph Whisnant of Rocky Mount Urology Associates, who after diagnosing me with prostate cancer, advised me to read and research as much as I possibly could on the subject. I made several trips to the library and various bookstores. I wrote several foundations and had them send me materials. I talked with individuals who were survivors of prostate cancer because they had caught the disease in time to adequately treat it. I also talked with those who sadly had waited too long to seek treatment and the disease had spread to other parts of their bodies. Having the appropriate information is the key to successfully battling prostate cancer.

Although writing this book required a great deal of time and effort on my part, it was not optional. Knowing what I now know about prostate cancer, I could not just go about my daily routine without any regard for the thousands of brothers who will be afflicted by this disease.

While writing this book, I literally had to go into seclusion from my congregation for days, instructing my wife, my administrative assistant, and church officers to only page me in case of emergency so I would have time to concentrate on the completion of this book. If sharing my experiences with prostate cancer can save just one life, then the energy I've exhausted in this effort is certainly worthwhile. I'm inclined to agree with Debra Harding who said, "thousands of lives will be saved as this book is read and put into practice."

Chapter 2

Only The Size Of A Walnut, But!!!

. . .a little member, and boasteth great things.
James 3:5

The question, "What is the prostate?" may seem simple to some readers. However, to men like myself, this question is one that never surfaced for the first forty years of my life. I would even venture to say that for most of my life, I never knew I had a prostate. I don't remember the prostate being one of the vital organs we studied in health class while in school.

Despite this ignorance that is unfortunately prevalent among many men, the prostate is a vital organ--the health of which can determine the quality of life, of loving and of personal liberty that most men hold dear to their hearts. Too often, men take for granted the vitality that a healthy prostate gives their whole being. My desire is to increase public awareness about this vital organ and to decrease the chances of a man not knowing what the prostate is until it is too late—when doctors tell him he has prostate cancer and that it has spread to other parts of his body.

The prostate is a walnut-sized gland located just below the bladder. It surrounds part of the urethra--the tube that carries urine from the bladder during urination. Its primary function is to provide fluid necessary for ejaculation.

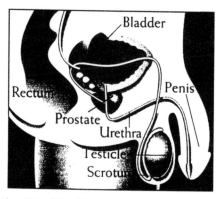

Illustration 2.1 - The Prostate and Surrounding Organs

If you are a male over age 40 and don't suffer from a prostate gland disorder, count your blessings. But not too fast. Chances are that as you age, you may begin to encounter urinary problems associated with an enlarged prostate.

In too many instances, common urinary problems such as: frequent urination, especially during the night; trouble starting the urine stream; and weak or interrupted urine stream; are considered a natural part of aging and are ignored for a significant period of time. The failure to attend to these symptoms will likely result in more severe prostate problems.

The three most common problems associated with the prostate are:

1. Infection
2. Enlargement
3. Growths

Infection

Infection usually starts in some other part of the body and spreads to the prostate. The infected prostate (a condition known as prostatitis) will swell and block the flow of urine through the urethra, which causes a backup in the bladder.

Acute prostatitis is a bacterial infection of the prostate. This condition is not age specific (It may occur at any age). Symptoms include fever, chills, and pain in the lower back and between the legs. This problem may cause pain or difficulty in urination. Treatment generally includes prescribing antibiotics and a recommendation that the patient drink more liquids.

Chronic prostatitis, on the other hand, is a recurring prostate infection. Although symptomatically similar to acute prostatitis, there is usually no fever. The symptoms are usually milder, but can last a long time. Chronic prostatitis is harder to treat because sometimes no disease-causing bacteria can be found. Antibiotics will generally work with bacteria infections. In some cases, doctors recommend warm baths or massaging the prostate to release fluids.

Prostate enlargement

Prostate enlargement is commonly called BPH or benign prostatic hyperplasia ("Benign" means the cells are non-cancerous, and "hyperplasia" means that there are more cells than normal). This condition is a result of growing older and, unfortunately, cannot be prevented. A man's chances of having this type of problem will increase as he becomes older.

BPH is symptomatic when accompanied by unpleasant urinary problems. One study estimates that half of the men in their 60's have BPH, and among men in their 70's and 80's, the figure may be as high as 90 percent. A man suffering from an enlarged prostate may have difficulty urinating, dribbling after urination and the urge to urinate often, especially at night. In some rare instances, the patient may be unable to urinate because the enlarged prostate may block the urethra. These same urinary symptoms are often shared by men with prostate cancer. Treatments for BPH may include:

- *Watchful waiting* - No treatment is given, but regular checkups are received. Both patient and doctor wait to see if the condition worsens. Your doctor may recommend this program if you are not bothered by your symptoms.

- *Alpha blockers* - These are drugs that help relax muscles near the prostate. They may relieve symptoms. Because these drugs are new, any effects of long-term usage are not known. Some known side effects may include headaches and dizziness.

- *Finasteride* (Proscar) - This is a drug that inhibits the action of the male hormone testosterone. It can shrink the prostate. Side effects include declining interest in sex, problems getting an erection, and problems with ejaculation. This drug is also new, so any long-term effects are not known.

- *Surgery* - This is most likely to relieve BPH symptoms, but it also has the most known complications. Three kinds of surgery are used for BPH treatment:

   1. Transurethral resection of the prostate (TURP) is the most common. The doctor inserts a special instrument into the urethra through the penis to remove part of the prostate to lessen its obstruction.

   2. Transurethral incision of the prostate (TUIP) may be used when the prostate is not too enlarged. The doctor passes an instrument through the urethra to make one or two small cuts in the prostate.

   3. Open surgery is used when the prostate is very enlarged. The doctor makes an incision in the abdomen or between the scrotum and the anus to remove prostate tissue.

Research continues to unveil new treatments for BPH every year. Examples include laser surgery, microwave thermal therapy, prostatic stents, and new drugs. Don't hesitate to ask for additional information if your doctor suggests any of these new methods.

Growths

Growths generally go undetected until they have spread beyond the most easily treated stage. Researchers say many men are living with prostate problems and don't even know it because the symptoms are so vague.

Mosby's Medical, Nursing, and Allied Health Dictionary defines prostate cancer as "a slowly progressive adenocarcinoma of the prostate gland that affects an increasing proportion of American males after the age of 50." Prostate cancer is one of the most common forms of cancer among American men. It remains a mystery why prostate cancer is more common among African American men than white men. In its early stages, prostate cancer stays in the prostate and is not life-threatening. But without treatment, it can metastasize (spread to other parts of the body).

Though serious, not all prostate cancers are equal. Some tumors may lie dormant for years, while others may be malignant and deadly. Size and appearance of the growth are some indications of its severity. Whether or not the disease has spread beyond the prostate itself is also an indication of the severity.

Through the use of PSA tests and ultra-sound guided biopsies, prostate cancer is more readily detectable. We men must take advantage of the opportunities afforded us through early detection and proper treatment.

Yes, my brothers, our prostates are only about the size of a walnut; however, a diseased prostate can be deadly. It is very important that every man over 40 have an annual checkup. A vital part of that physical should be a thorough examination of his prostate gland which should include a PSA (prostate specific antigen) test. The PSA numbers are critical numbers to know. A man over 40 years old should know his PSA as well as he knows his name, his social security number, or any other number. Some physicians may give you a digital rectal examination. In this examination, they use their finger to examine your prostate. This examination alone is inadequate to determine the true status of your prostate. My brother, insist that your doctor give you a PSA at least once a year.

Chapter 3

The Secret Storm

*Then he arose, and rebuked the wind and the raging of
the water: and they ceased, and there was a calm.*
Luke 8:24

Most of us are familiar with the old soap
opera, "The Secret Storm." In 1996, that phrase
literally became a reality for me. That's when I
was diagnosed with prostate cancer. Strangely
enough, when I discovered I had this dreadful
disease, I was in the midst of reading a book
entitled, "Preaching Through A Storm," by Dr. H.
Beecher Hicks, Jr. His book focuses on the pain
and predicament of preaching the gospel and
pastoring the 20th century congregation. In his
book, Dr. Hicks quotes William Augustus Jones,
Pastor of Bethany Baptist Church in Brooklyn,
New York, as saying the pastor is either "coming

out of a storm, in a storm, or heading for a storm." While I was reading the book to find out how to manage some unmanageable moments of my own ministry, little did I know I was really being prepared for a storm more major than any I had encountered in pastoring—the storm of prostate cancer.

One evening I was looking at a television program which had a panel of men discussing prostate cancer. The thought of going in for an examination crossed my mind, but I reasoned, "I'm only 46 and I feel great; so why worry about it." With my schedule, I don't get a chance to look at television often. But strangely enough, a few days later I stopped to look at television again. While scanning the channels, I ran across another interesting documentary about prostate cancer. It was becoming increasingly difficult for me to keep the thoughts of prostate problems out of my mind. But with my schedule, I soon found myself absorbed by the problems of others and my weekly regimen.

The thoughts, however, kept recurring. As I visited parishioners in the hospital, it seemed as though every male I visited made some reference to a prostate problem in himself or someone he knew. The silent struggle within me was at its peak, but it was still diluted by an almost dehumanizing schedule.

Several weeks later while waiting for my wife to complete her doctor visitation, I picked up a brochure containing an insert similar to this one.

	Yes	No
Do you urinate frequently, especially during the night?	❑	❑
Do you have trouble starting your urine stream?	❑	❑
Do you have a weak or interrupted urine stream?	❑	❑
Does it feel like your bladder isn't emptying completely?	❑	❑
Do you have blood in your urine?	❑	❑

Illustration 3.1

23

After reading this I realized that I had answered yes to at least two and maybe three of these questions. I thought, yes, I do urinate frequently especially during the night. Yes, I do have trouble starting my urine stream. And, as I think about it, yes I occasionally have a weak or interrupted urine stream. So I made an appointment with my urologist to get an examination.

My urologist talked with me about my concerns, asking the same questions posed on the brochure. After a brief conversation, he gave me a digital rectal exam. He stated that my prostate felt a little enlarged; however, a PSA test would be the thing to do to determine if there were any problems. A PSA (prostate specific antigen) is a blood test that measures a protein made only by the prostate. Prostate specific antigen is manufactured by the prostate and by cancerous cells within the prostate. An elevated PSA raises the possibility that cancer may be present. But I felt that there was not "a hint of a whisper, or a notion" that my PSA would be anything but normal. I was in for a surprise.

Following the PSA, my doctor said he would call my office with the lab results and/or send me a letter. He indicated that he did not expect any problems, but it's better to be safe than sorry. A few days later I received a letter from him suggesting that I come in for further tests because my PSA was 5.4. He went on to say that any count over 4.0 is unacceptable for a man my age. Needless to say, the storm was raging, but secretly.

When I returned to the urologist, he ordered a transrectal ultrasound (TRUS) and a biopsy. A transrectal ultrasound is a diagnostic procedure which uses a rectal probe to create an image of the prostate on a computer screen. The physician can then detect any abnormalities in the prostate. A biopsy is a simple surgical procedure in which a small piece of prostate tissue is removed with a needle and examined under a microscope to determine whether it is cancerous. Having these two tests behind me, I was faced with the most difficult time of all—the waiting period. My doctor still tried to reassure me that there may not be a serious problem. He pointed out that high PSAs could be an indication of prostatitis, a bacterial infection of the prostate, or benign prostatic hypertrophy (BPH), enlargement of the prostate. Both of these are noncancerous prostate problems. The doctor's reassurances lasted only temporarily. For, when the results came back, it was indeed cancerous. The sorrow and pain caused by the news was intensified because my wife was with me.

As you can imagine, the questions began to race through my mind. How can this be? I feel so good, how can this be happening to me? Why is this happening to me? What will happen to my family? What about my parishioners? There was such a flood of emotions and questions, and I wasn't quite sure what I needed to do.

Without a doubt, the day the doctor gave me the announcement that I had prostate cancer, truly was the darkest day I had ever experienced in my life. Yet, there was a rainbow in the midst of the dark clouds. I'm so thankful that I was able to be diagnosed in time. I'll say more about the importance of early diagnosis in the next chapter.

Not knowing then what I know now, it is hard to describe how I really felt. There was a kind of numbness that came all over me. It was almost as though a death sentence had been given me, and I was appointed to death row to await the time of execution. All of my past seemed fruitless, my present useless, and my future hopeless. I deeply regretted the fact that my wife was aware of my problem. I felt had she not known it, it could have really been my secret. I felt the need to be completely alone. I'm sure you remember the song of the 60's "Make the World Go Away." I wanted complete solitude and a chance to search my own soul for answers. Like Job of the Holy Scriptures, I wanted an audience with God to inquire why he allowed such tragedy in my life, after all of the work I had dedicated to his service. Clearly, the storm was raging and the billows were tossing high. But that was the down side.

The up side was that I began to appreciate the sunshine and rain, the flowers that bloom, and even the green grass more than ever before. I reasoned that I needed to spend more time with my grandchildren teaching them all I could about the virtues of life. I found myself gazing at them, saddened by the thought that I would probably be dead before they were teenagers. Another horrible thought was my wife, who was diagnosed with a degenerative neurological disorder, would possibly be faced with the problem of caring for me.

I never had a problem sleeping, but suddenly I found myself walking the floor in the wee hours of the morning--confused and full of questions. The storm was raging. Although I had encouraged others not to fear, my heart, mind and soul seemed engulfed by fear and anxiety. It seemed that my life was falling apart. Circumstances were out of control, and all I could do was pray. Then I thought of a song that I had produced several years earlier entitled "Down On My Knees." Some of the words of the song rang clearly in my mind:

When days are dark and friends are few
Lord, when I don't know just what to do
There's only one way I can find ease
I'll talk to Jesus down on my knees.

Down on my knees when trouble rise
I'll talk to Jesus beyond the skies
He promised me He'd hear my plea
If I just tell Him down on my knees.

And that I did! I'm convinced that we often *say* prayers in times of clear skies; but in the midst of a storm, we learn to *pray* prayers.

I thank God for my loving wife who, in spite of her own condition, encouraged me to draw upon my faith, to remember my own teaching and to continue to research the problem of prostate cancer. After she encouraged my heart through her thoughtful words, prayers, and concern, I remembered what "The Motivator" Les Brown said, "If life knocks you down, be sure to try and fall on your back because if you can look up, you can get up." I had recently ordered a set of his tapes. I recalled the powerful message he spoke on each of them. I listened, without ceasing, for several days at Les Brown's tapes. In fact, more than one night I was able to sleep only by wearing earphones with Les speaking to my inner conscience. I owe him much gratitude for the motivation his tapes provided me during my storm. I was shocked to hear that Les himself was stricken with prostate cancer, but I am pleased to hear that he sought appropriate treatment.

I intensified my prayers, sought answers through the Word of God, and read as many things as I could about the early detection and treatment of prostate cancer. I can truly say that any man who is faced with a traumatic announcement that he has prostate cancer needs to draw on all the resources he can find. Hopefully, he will have a loving and understanding family to support him and a strong faith in God to uphold him.

For years I had been known in the gospel world as "Mr. One Day At A Time," primarily because of a gospel recording I performed entitled, "One Day At A Time." Part of the chorus of that song says "Lord, for my sake, help me to take one day at a time." I would strongly advise anyone facing a similar problem to relax in God, try not to think the worst, ask questions of your doctor, quickly join a support group, and allow God to direct your path. Remember, He controls the storms and can say "Peace be still."

In spite of the advice just given, my storm was far from over. As you read the remaining chapters of this book, you will detect storms and calms, storms and calms, storms and calms. But I give God the glory for the calm moments produced by faith in His living Word, encouragement from loved ones, and power gained from absorbing knowledge about my condition. Knowing what I know now, I would strongly advise those of you who may find yourself confronted with the contrary winds of this dreadful disease not to struggle alone in the secret storm. Hopefully, the contents of this book will help to assure you that you don't have to weather the storm alone.

Chapter 4

Early Detection

My people are destroyed for lack of knowledge.
Hosea 4:6

Although I grew up in a single-parent home, I was blessed with the support and wisdom of a loving grandfather, who served as my male role model. My grandfather always taught me: ***It's better to be safe than sorry.*** This was never more true than with prostate cancer. Unfortunately, many men are not willing to go in for regular checkups and follow-ups with their urologists. It is definitely better to take the necessary precautionary steps--get regular checkups even though you may feel fine. Early detection of prostate cancer provides an excellent outlook for a complete cure. Undiagnosed and untreated, this disease proves fatal for thousands of men each year. Too many men are walking around with residual or metastasized prostate cancer when a simple visit with their urologist could save their lives.

Education is the first step to early detection. How much do you know about prostate cancer? Test your knowledge with the following "Prostate IQ Test."

Prostate IQ Test

True or False?

1. The prostate is a pear-shaped organ of the male reproductive system.

2. The main function of the prostate is to control the bladder.

3. A man's risk of developing prostate cancer at some time in his life is approximately 1 out of 100.

4. Early prostate cancer usually causes no symptoms.

5. The digital rectal exam should be performed only if you suspect prostate problems.

6. The basic prostate checkup is the x-ray of the prostate.

7. The PSA is a blood test used in the detection of prostate cancer.

8. An elevated PSA level is a definite indication that a patient has prostate cancer.

9. A biopsy is a type of treatment for cancer.

10. Cancer of the prostate is the most common form of malignancy in men.

11. Prostate cancer is the second leading cause of cancer deaths in men.

12. Prostate cancer accounts for 36% of all male cancers.

13. An oncologist is a doctor who specializes in surgery as a means of cancer treatment.

14. Not all prostate disease is cancerous.

15. Prostate cancer can usually be cured if it is treated before the disease spreads.

(Turn to page 40 to check your answers.)

If you answered at least 14 items correctly, you have managed to stay abreast of the current research related to prostate disease. If you answered 10-13 items correctly, you are fairly knowledgeable about prostate disease. If you answered less than 10 items correctly, I strongly recommend that you read as much as you can about the subject.

If you are diagnosed with prostate cancer, it is extremely important that you understand how far it has advanced. Prostate cancer is classified in stages: A, B, C, or D. The outlook for successful treatment is dependent upon the stage at diagnosis. The following chart shows the stages of development and the characteristics of each stage. Even the selection of the appropriate treatment will be based upon the stage of prostate cancer.

Stages of Prostate Cancer	
Stage	**Characteristics**
A	Confined to prostate, not felt during digital rectal exam
B	Confined to prostate, diagnosed by digital rectal exam
C	Has grown beyond prostate into neighboring tissues
D	Has spread to the pelvic lymph nodes or to more distant parts of the body, such as the bones

*Digital rectal exams are not sufficient to detect all prostate cancer. It is very important that you request a **PSA** as a part of the examination given by your urologist.*

Illustration 4.1

If diagnosis occurs while the disease is confined to the prostate and prompt treatment follows, a patient is generally successfully treated. On the other hand, if the disease has reached stage D, the average survival period is only about three years. The American Cancer Society and the

National Cancer Institute indicated in 1997 that 53%-59% of prostate cancer cases were localized (clinical stages A and B), 13%-18% were regional (clinical stage C), and 11%-20% were metastatic (clinical stage D) at the time of diagnosis.

Equally as important as education is the need for regular medical checkups that include a prostate examination. Even if you have had surgery for BPH, you are not exempt from prostate cancer. Any remaining part of your prostate is subject to cancer. The odds of early detection are increased dramatically with the introduction of the prostate specific antigen (PSA) test. If a man's prostate becomes enlarged or damaged, it may release increased amounts of PSA. This test alone cannot determine whether a man has cancer, but it does alert a doctor that a potential problem exists with the prostate.

When elevated PSAs are present, doctors will generally follow-up with a transrectal ultrasound (TRUS), using a rectal probe to create a video image of the prostate, and/or a biopsy, taking a tiny tissue sample from the prostate. No anti-cancer treatment of any kind should be employed until it is definitively established that the patient has prostate cancer.

As of March 1998, a new PSA was approved by the FDA called the free PSA. It measures the amount of free floating PSA in the blood, and can help determine whether men with elevated PSA levels should even get biopsies (Richmond Times-Dispatch, Thursday, June 4, 1998).

Certain men are at greater risk of getting prostate cancer. They include:

- Men over age 50. However, 80% of prostate cancer is diagnosed in men over 65.

- African Americans, who have a 66% increased risk for prostate cancer.

- Those with a family history of prostate cancer.

You owe it to yourself, your family, and your friends to protect yourself against this potentially deadly disease. Be sure! Do it for those who love you.

Answers to Prostate IQ Test
1. **F**; 2. **F**; 3. **F**; 4. **T**; 5. **F**
6. **F**; 7. **T**; 8. **F**; 9. **F**; 10. **T**
11. **T**; 12. **T**; 13. **F**; 14. **T**; 15. **T**

Chapter 5

The Big "C"

Yea, though I walk through the valley of the shadow of
death, I will fear no evil: for thou art with me;
thy rod and thy staff they comfort me.
Psalm 23:4

In my twenty-seven years of pastoring I had
seen many cancer cases among my parishioners
and friends. I had counseled men, women and
children after they had been told that their bodies
had been invaded by this terrible disease. I had
listened with interest while in fervent prayer as
they pondered over their method of treatment.
Would it be surgery? Radiation? Chemotherapy?
Or just do nothing? Needless to say, I had seen
too many of them waste away in a sometimes
painful death regardless of the options they chose.
This was frightening. In my mind, cancer was

cancer whether it be lung cancer, breast cancer, skin cancer, colon cancer, etc. In my mind, cancer was the equivalent of death.

Many people feel the same way. Some feel that cancer and hope are not bed partners. Others feel that treatments for cancer have the same side effects regardless of the type of cancer and where it is located. I was talking with a friend who had a very low PSA count, but his biopsy showed that he had cancer cells. This friend was over 65 years old and could have possibly been spared a lot of pain and discomfort as well as the side effects of incontinence and complete impotence. But one year prior to my even knowing what he was experiencing, he had a radical prostatectomy. Once I found out what had happened, I asked him why he hadn't chosen radiation as a treatment. His reply was, "I've seen what happens to people who take radiation, how their hair comes out and their skin color changes. I just didn't want that to happen to me." Clearly, there are some misunderstandings about treatments and their side effects and we will address them in future chapters.

Let's return to my urologist's office and tune in to the conversation between us after he told me I had prostate cancer. Your urologist can literally make or break you if you are so unfortunate to be told you have prostate cancer. If he or she insists on just being a physician and not a friend and perhaps a counselor, your road will be both fearful and uncertain. My doctor continued to encourage me by saying he felt we were ahead of the problem. He also comforted my wife as she sat with me in that treatment room that seemed to have been closing in on both of us. However, I was wondering if I needed to even listen to him. After all, this was the same fellow who told me after the digital rectal examination that it could just be an enlarged prostate. After the PSA this same fellow told me that the high reading could be just a result of some benign infection. Now that I know I have cancer this same fellow is telling me I need to go to Nash

General Hospital and take a bone scan to see if the prostate cancer has metastasized (spread beyond the original site of the tumor). "But," he added, "I feel certain that it has not because of the low PSA count and the size and location of the cancer cells." The question in my mind was should I join in his optimism now when his earlier optimistic expectations proved to be futile. But in retrospect, had he not coached me through each step I would have surely lost hope and possibly made the wrong decisions.

He made an appointment for me to have a bone scan. He explained that the purpose of the test was to see if the cancer cells had spread beyond the original site into the bones and lymph nodes. This too was a challenge for me because of the uncertainty of the outcome. In addition, I have trouble with claustrophobia; the idea of lying still for a long period of time while they scanned my body was very uncomfortable to me.

The staff at Nash General Hospital was very helpful in assuring me that the process would only take about 45 minutes. They gave me an injection and told me to go back home for about two hours and drink plenty of water. I found out later that the injection was a radioactive substance that went throughout my body and settled especially into my bone structure.

When I returned to the hospital, they scanned my body slowly from my head to my toes. The nurse informed me that if there was a bone area infected with cancer, it would tend to absorb more of the radiation material than the normal bone. I told her to take her time and look as carefully as possible because by now I discovered through my reading that if the cancer had escaped, my treatment options were lessened and much more critical.

After each test was performed, there was a waiting period for the results. I can say in no uncertain terms that those were the longest days of my life. The storm was not over. Each day literally seemed like a month. About five days after the bone scan, my doctor's nurse called my office and asked me to come by to discuss the results. As my doctor walked in the treatment room, he had a smile on his face and said , "I'm happy to tell you the test showed no spread of the cancer beyond the prostate." That was a great time of joy and calm.

Release from the fear of the worst will certainly heip you feel better about what you're going through. After getting that report and having done a lot of reading and research, I felt much better about my prognosis. My research showed that once the cancer spreads beyond the prostate and gets into the bones it could end up in any part of your body, such as your legs, your lymph nodes, your liver, etc. I also found that prostate cancer out of control can lead to a very painful death. I felt extremely blessed that the bone scan was negative.

For several days I was on a high from the good news that the cancer had not spread beyond the prostate and metastasized. It's hard to explain the joy I felt as a result of that good news. However, a few days later I woke up very depressed because the reality of my still having "The Big C" overwhelmed me. I knew that something had to be done, but what?

I shall never forget my encounter with my good friend, The Rev. Jesse Jackson. Jesse called me and asked me to meet him at a labor union rally in eastern North Carolina. As I sat on the platform at the rally listening to Jesse's usual eloquent speaking and noticing how engrossed the audience was with his message, several thoughts crossed my mind. I thought, he is such a giving person, always traveling throughout the world serving this present age. I wonder if he's getting his prostate checked as he should. I wonder what is his PSA reading. I started to ask him about it at the conclusion of the rally, but decided the timing was not right.

Jesse quickly called another meeting with the ministers in an adjacent building. In that meeting he was giving out assignments, as only Rev. Jesse Jackson can do. He asked me to chair an effort for the Rainbow Coalition; and although I consented, little did he know of the secret storm still raging in my mind. You see, I had not told Jesse about my condition. Quite frankly, I owe Jesse an apology because I never carried out that assignment. I was so overwhelmed about the uncertainty of my future until I was preoccupied with research and meditation. I do not wish the announcement of cancer of any form on anyone. However, the remaining chapters of this book will attest to the fact that there can be life after the Big "C."

Chapter 6

My Medical Records

Ye shall know the truth and the truth
shall make you free.
John 8:32

In an effort to be as transparent as possible about this serious disease that has taken the lives of so many men in America, I am revealing portions of my medical records. My heart's desire is that there will be no doubt in anyone's mind that prostate cancer was a reality in my life. Through the blessings of God and the insistence of Dr. Joseph Whisnant, my urologist, and Dr. Samuel Wesonga, my personal physician, I am cured. Because of the patience of these two doctors, I was introduced to Dr. Frederick Ellwanger, radiologist at Nash General Hospital who provided significant orientation on brachytherapy, and Dr. Jerrold Sharkey, the physician who treated me with brachytherapy. (This procedure will be discussed later.)

The following documents were taken directly from my medical files. These documents not only authenticate my bout with cancer, but also reveal how difficult I was as a patient.

General Checkup
No Real Concerns

ROCKY MOUNT UROLOGY ASSOCIATES. P.A.
PROGRESS NOTES

WALKER, REV. THOMAS
#34396
11-27-95

S: Rev. Walker has been followed here with stone disease in the past
and comes today without clinical symptoms, but at age 47 would like a
check of his prostate and PSA. We discussed this at some length. He
has no family history of prostate cancer. His voiding pattern is stable
and normal. He has not had any definite stone disease, although an
episode of red urine some years ago that may have represented passage of
a small calculus. He was treated with ESWL in 1989, and a film in 1993
by Dr. Macaulay showed no definite stones. There may have been a tiny
stone in the upper pole on the right side on that film, but this is a
nebulous finding. It may or may not still be present on KUB today.

O: His UA is completely clear. On rectal exam, prostate is 20-25
grams and is broad, flat, and benign. The KUB shows a questionable 3-mm
stone in upper pole of the right kidney. This is a vague finding.

A: 1.   Calcium oxalate urolithiasis metabolically and surgically
inactive at present.
     2.   Prostate exam revealing some findings consistent with BPH,
but normal exam.

P: A PSA is obtained. We will write a report. As long as it is
stable, routine follow-up in 12 months is suggested. Force fluids in an
attempt to prevent further stone difficulties.
JDW/PTS-dw

Illustration 6.1

First Red Flag
Signs of Concern

ROCKY MOUNT UROLOGY ASSOCIATES. P.A.
PROGRESS NOTES

NAME: *Thomas L. Walker*   CHART#: 34396   DATE: 12-18-96

S: Rev. Walker is back in after I sent him a letter noting that his PSA is increased for age. His value is 5.46. This is his initial PSA value he is just 50 at this time. He has a quite large prostate on DRE but is completely benign and I strongly suspect that this is the source of the elevation. I brought him back, however, for a prostate massage to assess for infection and to discuss with him the various options that are available including the ultrasound and biopsy which I think should be considered simply based on the PSA value. Note that he has no history of prostate cancer in the family. His father had fairly significant prostatism and BPH and I believe that I cared for him here surgically.

O: His urinalysis is completely clear and on rectal exam the prostate is 20 to 30 grams and it is massaged and there is no induration. Mild to moderate tenderness. The EPS are basically clear.

A: Marginal to increased PSA for age with normal DRE and significant BPH by DRE.

P: 1.   I have asked him to repeat a PSA in approximately 1 week and I offered him ultrasound and biopsy and I have discussed 3 separate options one of which would be to simply follow him and recheck PSA in 6 months to 12 months hoping that this is simply his baseline value and suspect that it is.

2.   Proceed directly with ultrasound and biopsy and I have told him in honesty that this is the only way to exclude prostate malignancy. Although it does not completely do so, it is the only definite test. A third option which we discussed would be to simply obtain a PSA density with the ultrasound. I told him that this does not guarantee against malignancy but would be reassuring if the value is less than 0.15. He would like to go slowly with this process and it not anxious to proceed directly with biopsy and I have therefore made him an appointment again in 2 weeks after he has the PSA repeated and we will make some decisions then about how to proceed.

JDW/jgf

Illustration 6.2

Follow-Up Visit
More Tests Needed

ROCKY MOUNT UROLOGY ASSOCIATES. P.A.
PROGRESS NOTES

NAME: *Rev. Walker* CHART#: *34396* DATE: *1·10·96*

```
WALKER, THOMAS
#34396
1/10/96
```

S: Rev. Walker is back today in follow-up. His repeat PSA was 5.31, basically unchanged from the previous value. I have discussed with him at length the options that have been offered which include 1) biopsy, 2) ultrasound exam and PSA density calculation, 3) simple observation and repeat PSA. Of these three options, I would favor going ahead with ultrasound and biopsy in this young man to exclude the possibility of carcinoma. I have told him, however, that I think statistically the odds are quite strong in his favor and that the likelihood is that this simply represents his baseline related to a large prostate. He understands, however, that the only true test is a biopsy of the prostate that would exclude carcinoma. I have explained the risks of the test with particular reference to infection or even urosepsis and bleeding that could occur from prostate biopsies. I think he understands this risk and accepts it well and wishes to proceed with ultrasound and biopsy. We will schedule this for him in the next several weeks.

A: Increased PSA with normal DRE. Rule out occult prostatic carcinoma.

P: 1. Ultrasound and biopsies to be scheduled at his convenience.
  2. Regular prep with preoperative antibiotics and enema.
JDW/PTS-1e

Illustration 6.3

Follow-up Visit
Cautious Optimism

ROCKY MOUNT UROLOGY ASSOCIATES. P.A.
PROGRESS NOTES

WALKER, REV. THOMAS
#34396
1/19/96

S: Rev. Walker is back today in follow-up. Ultrasound and biopsy of
his prostate is accomplished. The gland is moderately large measuring
about 43 cc in volume by ultrasound measurement. PSA density calculate
using the value of 5.31 for PSA is within acceptable range at 0.1223.
There was, however, a hypoechoic area that was seen fairly discrete in
the central/transition zone which was well localized, and two cores of
tissue were taken from this area. A single core from the base on the
left and a core from the midportion and towards the apex on the right
are obtained with no significant bleeding or hematoma.

A: PSA increase in a 47-year-old gentleman. Rule out carcinoma.

P: 1.   Cipro 500 mg po on a b.i.d. schedule.
      2.   Routine follow-up here in a week for reports.
      3.   He knows to call or return immediately if he develops any
fever, bleeding, pain, voiding symptoms, or other problems related to
the procedure.
JDW/PTS-1e

Illustration 6.4

The Day The Bomb Dropped

ROCKY MOUNT UROLOGY ASSOCIATES. P.A.
PROGRESS NOTES

WALKER, REV. THOMAS
#~~39203~~ #34396
1-24-96

S: Rev. Walker is back in today, and unfortunately I had to give him the diagnosis of adenocarcinoma of the prostate. He has a moderately differentiated tumor in the left lobe of his prostate that was a Gleason 5 on histologic exam. Two cores were involved, and I think the hypoechoic area that we could see fairly deep in the central portion of the prostate is the tumor itself. I have told him that I certainly hope that this is a localized tumor, and based on our data presently, would presume that it is. His clinical stage I think would be T2B NXMX at present. We had a very lengthy discussion of treatment options which would include radical prostatectomy, radiation therapy, hormonal therapy, or observation. I told him that I would favor either surgical therapy or radiation therapy, and that I think in a man his age who is otherwise in good health that probably the surgical approach with radical prostatectomy would be most appropriate. He asked a number of intelligent questions about the disease. His wife was present at the conference. I gave him the literature recently published from the AUA with recommendations for localized prostate cancer, and also recommended that he purchase a copy of Dr. Patrick Walch's book on the prostate, which I think has excellent information in detail about options that are available to him along with statistical data that would help him make decisions. He is somewhat taken aback with this diagnosis, and I think he wants to think about this at some length.

A: Clinical stage T2B NXMX adenocarcinoma of the prostate.

P: An acid phosphatase is drawn today. I have suggested we go ahead with a bone scan. He would like to wait on this for the next several weeks. I have told him I think we should not procrastinate for any length of time, but I think it would be reasonable to seek another opinion if he would so desire. We would be glad to help him find this. He is to call us to schedule the bone scan, and then once this information is available, we will let it be known. He would like us to call him the acid phosphatase result, and I will do so just as soon as it is available to us.
JDW/PTS-dw
cc: Dr. Samuel Wesonga

Illustration 6.5

Follow-up Visit
What To Do When You Don't Know What To Do

ROCKY MOUNT UROLOGY ASSOCIATES. P.A.
PROGRESS NOTES

WALKER, REV. THOMAS
#34396
08-12-96

S: Rev. Walker is back today to again discuss therapy. He has been treating himself
alternative medicine for his prostate tumor, we have advised against this and again
discussed it today. I have told him that I think he really should strongly consider
surgical therapy again as his best option. He would like to have his PSA repeated, wan
me to repeat an ultrasound to recheck his prostate but has agreed to allow me to try to
make a time for a consultation with Dr. Patrick Walsh. I told him that I think Dr. Wal
is I think indeed the best surgeon in the country to do this particular procedure and I
would like him to least talk with him to get his advice about what is most appropriate.
have told him that the wait may be several months in doing this, he understands this bu
willing to proceed at least this far. Accordingly, I will contact Dr. Walsh as soon as
possible and try to make a time to have him seen in the near future, at least for
consultation and consideration of surgical therapy.

O: His prostate feels benign on exam, there might be slight thickening in the right l
although basically it is a normal exam. Note the fact that on a good dietary control a
low fat diet he has lost 20-30 pounds since he was last here, this has been I think on
own initiative.

A: Adenocarcinoma of the prostate, ? progressive, clinical Stage T2B.

P: 1. PSA is repeated.
2. We will schedule an ultrasound in the near future.
3. I will contact Dr. Patrick Walsh as soon as possible for an appointment for
consultation at Hopkins in Baltimore.
JDW:TTS/mb

Illustration 6.6

Telephone Conversation
Dr. Joseph Whisnant
A persistent, loving physician

ROCKY MOUNT UROLOGY ASSOCIATES. P.A.
PROGRESS NOTES

WALKER, REV. THOMAS
#34396
8-16-96

PHONE CONVERSATION: I called Dr. Patrick Walsh who is Professor of Urologic Surgery at the Brady Urologic Institute of Johns Hopkins University and who is generally considered to be one of the finest prostate surgeons in the country and the man who devised the potency-sparing operation. I presented Rev. Walker's case to him and asked if he would see him in an attempt to discuss with him possible surgical therapy as Rev. Walker and I had discussed here in the office on his recent visit. Dr. Walsh said that he would be glad to talk with him but that he would not convince him of his need for surgery. He felt that if he had made a decision against surgery and it was well informed that he should be allowed to do so. He felt that the best we can do in situations where we feel that surgery is the best option would be to advise the patient and then we must accept the decision made. I agree with this entirely but would at least like Rev. Walker to have at one more opportunity to talk with someone who is extremely knowledgeable about the disease. He said that he would see him if he would call and make an appointment. Accordingly I will write Rev. Walker a letter with Dr. Walsh's phone number and recommend to him that he go ahead and make an appointment. Note that his PSA has returned in the 9 range.

JDW:TTS/mb

(signature) Whisnant

Illustration 6.7

Follow-up Visit
A Feeling Of Desperation
Now, I must seek medical treatment

ROCKY MOUNT UROLOGY ASSOCIATES. P.A.
PROGRESS NOTES

NAME: _Rev. Thomas Walker_ CHART#:_____ DATE: _8-28-96_

S: Rev. Walker comes back today for repeat US of his prostate. I think that the lesion in his prostate that we suspect as the primary tumor appears to have increased some in size. This is not dramatic but his PSA has increased significantly almost doubling in the last 6 to 8 months. He has been thinking about this and has decided that he wants to proceed with radiation therapy. I had felt that surgery would be better for this young man but he is extremely concerned about potency and issues of complications related to radical prostatectomy. I had strongly suggested to him and recommended to him that he see Dr. Patrick Walsh at Hopkins in Baltimore for his assessment and recommendations. He has decided that he does not want to do this but is willing to go ahead and be treated at this time with radiation therapy. I think that perhaps this would be my second choice but am quite happy that he has agreed to undergo treatment at this point. Accordingly, I discussed with him again all of the treatment options including cryotherapy and brachii therapy. He wishes to proceed with external beam irradiation and I will make contact with Dr. Elwanger and/or Dr. Connell to arrange to have him seen as soon as possible. NOTE that he has some microscopic blood in his urine today. He has had stone disease in the past and I suspect that this is etiologic. Rather than push him towards cysto which I do not believe that he wants at this point, I think that we can get good images of his kidneys with the CT scans and if we can confirm stone disease at some point and endoscopic exam of his bladder would be appropriate to exclude disease in the lower tract. I have made an appointment for him in 6 to 8 weeks and would hope to be able to do this or at least schedule it around that time.

Illustration 6.8

Follow-up Visit
Check Me One More Time

RADIOLOGICAL CONSULTATION

Thomas Walker
34396
8-28-96
Prostate ultrasound
JDW

Ultrasound of the prostate is accomplished again at Rev. Walker's request to assess his prostate tumor. He has elected against any therapy since the diagnosis was made some 7 to 8 months ago of prostate carcinoma. His PSA has increased and I have told him that we would be glad to repeat the test to help him make a decision about treatment. Accordingly, the seminal vesicles are imaged at the base and they are somewhat thickened, symmetrical and normal and unchanged from his previous ultrasound. The base of the prostate, midportion at 3 levels and apex, is then imaged. The margins of the prostate are somewhat irregular but towards the midportion on the left side is an area that is hypoechoic down in the central portion of the prostate that I think has increased somewhat in size when it is compared with his old films. This is the area that was positive on needle biopsy. The area measures greater than 2 cm in size at this point. It still appears to be confined to the prostate although I do not think that this can be ascertained from ultrasound exam.

I: Comparative ultrasound is obtained after a diagnosis of moderately differentiated adenocarcinoma has been made. The lesion suspect as the primary tumor in this gentleman appears to have increased somewhat in size although the volume increased is fairly minimal. Note that PSA is increased from the 5 range to the 9 range, I think, indicating significant tumor activity. Treatment has been recommended to him.

JDW/jgf

Rocky Mount Urology Associates

Joseph D. Whisnant, M.D.
Gordon L. Mathes, M.D.
Robert B. Whitmore, III, M.D.
Frederick A. Frohbose, M.D.
180 Foy Drive
Rocky Mount, NC 27804
443-3136

Illustration 6.9

Referral to Radiologist
A Hard-headed Patient

August 30, 1996

Frederick Ellwanger, M. D.
Department of Radiation Oncology
Nash Day Hospital
2450 Curtis Ellis Drive
Rocky Mount NC 27804

RE: REVEREND THOMAS WALKER
RMU# 34396

Dear Rick:

This is to introduce Reverend Thomas Walker. I saw him for routine screening of his prostate in January of this year and have followed him in the past for intermittent stone disease. At the time we saw him his PSA was slightly elevated and after repeating the test and reexamining him, we felt that for a 47 year old man the value of 5.46 despite a large prostate was not acceptable and recommended to him that he undergo needle biopsies. This was accomplished on 01-19-96. A volume of his prostate was 43 cc, the PSA at that time was 5.31 with a PSA density that would have been in the acceptable range at 0.122. There was a fairly discreet area that was hypoechoic however in the central/transition zone in the left anterior prostate. Two biopsies were taken from this area and unfortunately have shown Gleason V moderately differentiated adenocarcinoma, clinical stage of his disease would be T2A, ? T2BNXM0, his bone scan was negative. discussed with him on several occasions, in the presence of his wife, the findings and told him that I think in a man his age that the best option would be radical prostatectomy. Given the complications that are possible with this procedure, particularly with loss of sexual function he was very much opposed to the same and then disappeared from our office here. recommended that he get a second opinion, he asked that I send him to the urologist in Greenville, Dr. Greg Murphy, who saw him and recommended think essentially the same. I offered him visits to the local medical centers or to Dr. Patrick Walsh at Hopkins but he preferred instead to treat his disease with dietary restrictions and with herbs. He has lost about 20-30 pounds on this diet in the last 4-6 months and Dr. Sam Wesonga is his personal physician who has looked after him through this. He was back

requesting that we repeat his PSA and an ultrasound, I think hoping that the disease would be stable or perhaps relenting. Unfortunately, the lesion has increased in size I think, at least somewhat, and his PSA has gone from the 5 range to 9.58.

Illustration 6.10

Referral to Radiologist

(page 2 of 2)

We discussed this at some length in the office yesterday. I discussed all of the treatment options again with him including brachytherapy and cryotherapy although we feel that these are peripheral treatments at present. He has elected to go with radiation therapy and is to the point now that he feels that he needs to be treated. I think that this is a better solution certainly than no treatment in his particular case and would appreciate very much if you would see him, talk with him, and if you are in agreement that radiation therapy is appropriate treatment for him, then obtain a CT scan for appropriate treatment planning, as well as, CT scans of his kidneys as microscopic hematuria was noted on this visit and he has a history of stone disease. This will image his upper tracts and at a later time we can accomplish further examination of his bladder if it is felt necessary. At this point, I think the primary directive should be to get treatment for his diagnosed and known prostate cancer. If you will simply call his office at 446-2378 or home at 442-4244 and make him a convenient appointment, we would greatly appreciate it.

Sincerely,

Joseph D. Whisnant, Jr., M. D.

JDW:TTS/mb

CC: Dr. Wesonga

Chapter 7

An African American Perspective

*So teach us to number our days, that we may apply
our hearts unto wisdom.*
Psalm 90:12

Fact or fiction? African Americans comprise one-third of America's poor. Fact or fiction? African Americans have lower educational attainment. Fact or fiction? African Americans have poorer access and availability to quality health care. Unfortunately, all of the above statements are fact. Many experts believe that these and other factors contribute to the disproportionate number of cancer cases in the African American community.

The effects of prostate cancer in the African American community are far-reaching. Most African Americans have a friend or relative who is either living with the disease or one who has died from it. The incidence of prostate cancer in the African American community has doubled in the past 25 years. African American males are more likely to get this disease, and they are more likely to develop it at an earlier age. More than 6,000 African American men die each year from prostate cancer.

According to statistical data presented to the Subcommittee on National Security House Committee on Appropriations in March 1998 by Jay H. Hedlund (President and CEO of the National Prostate Cancer Coalition), "African Americans have the highest prostate cancer incidence in the world. Incidence rates are 66 percent higher for African Americans than Caucasian men and mortality rates are more than two times higher." To review the entire document "Testimony Of The National Prostate Cancer

Coalition, Jay H. Hedlund, President and CEO," contact:

> National Prostate Cancer Coalition
> 1156 15th Street, NW, Suite 905
> Washington, DC 20005
> Tel: (202) 463-9455
> Fax: (202) 463-9456
> www.dnpcc.org

Jay Hedlund gives high accolades to Robert Samuels, Chairman of the National Prostate Cancer Coalition and a prostate cancer survivor. "Bob Samuels. . . has been a dedicated and effective advocate in the fight to finally find a cure for prostate cancer. His caring and unflagging commitment has helped NPCC make real inroads in the fight to secure adequate federal funding for prostate cancer research that will lead to a cure for this devastating disease." Without a doubt, Bob's assistance has been invaluable in my quest to secure information.

The statistics provided by the American Cancer Society are staggering.

- African Americans have the highest overall cancer incidence of any ethnic or racial group in America.

- African Americans have the highest mortality rates of any ethnic or racial group in America.

- African Americans are less likely than whites to survive cancer five years after diagnosis.

- African Americans are more likely to be diagnosed at a later stage of the disease.

- African American smokers have a higher incidence of smoking-related illnesses than white smokers because they smoke more and are more likely to smoke higher tar and nicotine brands of cigarettes.

- African Americans tend to eat foods higher in fat and engage in relatively less regular physical activity.

The Society cites several issues it believes contribute to the higher incidences of cancer:

- Tobacco use
- Poor nutrition
- Insufficient physical activity
- Inadequate access to screening, early diagnosis and treatment

Although cancer knows no racial or ethnic boundaries, it is obvious that African Americans are over-represented when we look at the number of cancer victims. Research indicates that socio-economic factors, such as educational attainment, income and availability to quality health care have a direct impact on cancer incidences, mortality, and survival.

Facts and Figures

The following facts and figures will give us some indication of why cancer incidences and deaths are so prevalent in the African American community.

<u>Population</u>

- African Americans comprise the largest minority group in America.

- In 1990, African Americans numbered nearly 30 million and constituted 12% of the U.S. population.

- Between 1980 and 1990, the African American population increased by about 4 million.

- The majority of African Americans in the United States are descendants of slaves from Africa.

- In 1990, 54% of African Americans lived in the South, 18% lived in the Northeast, 19% lived in the Midwest and 9% lived in the West; 84% of African Americans lived in Metropolitan areas.

- The majority of the African American population is young. In 1990, about 77% were under age 45, and of those 33% were under age 18. Only 8% were 65 or older.

Family Structure

- In 1992 only 50% of African American families were married-couple families.

- The proportion of African American children who lived with just one parent increased from 32% in 1970 to 55% in 1990 (a 72% increase)

Income

- The mid-range income for African American families was approximately $22,000 in 1989.

- Income is strongly related to family structure, showing a $20,000 increase in married families.

- African Americans earn less money than their white counterparts and are more likely to live in poverty.

- Since 1960, the median family income has remained about 60% of the median family income for white families.

Health Status

The lower socio-economic status quite often leads to the unavailability of health care. African Americans generally have poorer insurance coverage, thus making quality health care inaccessible.

There appears to be a direct correlation between socio-economic status and knowledge of appropriate health care, attitudes concerning proper health care, and behaviors concerning health matters. Individuals with lower socio-economic status are generally more difficult to recruit for screening and other health service programs. They are also more likely to delay in seeking appropriate medical attention.

What Can Be Done?

Education is the key. There must be increased efforts to provide information targeted to the African American citizen. The education should stress lifestyle changes to include:

- a healthy diet
- an exercise program
- early cancer screening

- avoiding smoking
- a greater willingness to participate in
  clinical research trials

Health care must also be accessible and affordable. If access to early diagnosis and treatment of cancer were provided to all low-income and uninsured Americans, it would substantially reduce the cancer mortality rate in African Americans and in all Americans.

It is my prayer that this book will serve as a major educational tool, especially in the African American community. I trust religious organizations will assist in pointing out the urgent need of more education in the African American community. There must be a conscious effort to educate our people through whatever means necessary. I believe the church will be our greatest avenue for reaching our people.

Chapter 8

I'll Fix It

...herb for the service of man.
Psalm 105:14

Several years ago, I had an opportunity to attend a seminar being sponsored by a local hospital for the purpose of training pastors in the volunteer chaplain program. I never shall forget the opening words of the keynote speaker when he said we need to be sensitive to those patients to whom we have been called to minister. We need to understand what they are faced with. Ninety-eight percent of the time, people doctor on themselves. If they have a headache, they take an Excedrin. If they have a muscle ache, they rub down in Ben Gay. If they have a stomach ache, they take an Alka Seltzer, or perhaps even the old home remedy of baking soda. If they have a backache, they may take a Doan's pill. Ninety-eight percent of the time, they're able to do whatever is necessary to take care of the problem. It's only two percent of the time that they find themselves at a point when they have to give themselves over to the care of a physician and possibly a hospital stay. Just that thought alone may make them feel helpless, powerless, and frustrated.

Needless to say, on the day my doctor told me I had prostate cancer, I sensed those feelings more than ever before. The emotions that went through me were just multiplied. I felt doubt (Is it true?) Secondly, could the doctor have made a mistake? How could something so serious be wrong with me when I had little or no symptoms? Can something this serious happen to a 47 year old man who has always been in generally good health? The doctors say this is a slow growing cancer, maybe I can out-maneuver it. Maybe I can reverse the process of these "out-of-control" cells called cancer.

I'LL FIX IT!!!

I wasn't ready to give myself over to the conventional medical procedures. In fact, to be honest, I had all kinds of negative thoughts about the motives of my urologist and the entire conventional medical community. Is surgery or radiation, or any other conventional treatment really necessary to rid me of this problem? . . . If in fact, I truly have a problem? If I resort to natural remedies, could they deliver me? I had always said if I were ever stricken with a terminal disease, I would make some new discoveries by trying every natural remedy known to man until I was cured. Well, my greatest fears had become a reality. However, I believed that through prayer and natural home remedies, I could beat the odds.

My first goal was to enter into an intensive cleansing program that I had heard a friend talk about. This was a 10-day fasting process combined with cleansing my digestive system. Simultaneous to the intensive cleansing, I engaged in a process of juicing fruit and vegetables, consuming fruit juice in the morning and vegetable juice in the evening. Also, I was in a rigid exercise program followed up by long periods of lying in the sun, expecting health benefits from its energies.

It was obvious to those around me that something strange was going on in my life. I dropped from a weight of 218 lbs. to 168 lbs. I felt great and many of my friends said in my presence that I looked great. But I later learned, that was their public opinion. Their private opinion was that I had something bad, and that I was swiftly wasting away. The rumors ranged from my having AIDS to an acute case of diabetes. But I was determined that I would fix it. In retrospect, I discovered that while a reasonable health maintenance program is always in order, my intensive regimen was anything but reasonable. In fact, it was radical and life-threatening. I thank God I quit while I was ahead.

Currently, there is a strong debate about the merits of conventional medicine as opposed to natural medicine. Quite frankly, both have their place in preventing and fighting the dreadful disease--cancer. Certainly, no one can deny the benefits of a healthy lifestyle--eating right, exercising properly, and generally taking care of your body.

Research indicates that certain minerals, vitamins and chemicals can help combat cancer cells. Antioxidants, vitamins A, C, and E, and selenium have also become topics of debate. The debate is not over whether they have nutritional value, but rather whether they are therapeutic in nature.

Studies show that Vitamin E is very effective in preventing and treating prostate cancer. The question is continuously asked, "Are large doses of these nutritional supplements beneficial in the treatment of cancer?" Advocates for natural medicine believe the public should be made aware of potentially life-saving alternatives. On the other hand, the opponents of natural medicine will strongly argue against claims of natural healing, stating that large doses of these nutritional supplements are costly and that excessive doses may, in fact, create other health problems. If you or someone you love is diagnosed with prostate cancer, you owe it to yourself to investigate every possible treatment option.

I tried every nutritional remedy I could find. I'm sure I was helped by them, but it wasn't lowering my PSA count. In fact, during my rigorous nutritional regimen, my PSA level increased. I later discovered that the critical difference in prostate cancer and some other cancers is that prostate cancer feeds on testosterone, while several other cancers are positively affected by the boosting of the immune system.

Upon going to my family physician for a complete physical and blood tests of all sorts, including a PSA, I was given a clean bill of health with all other portions of the examination except my PSA. It had moved in a matter of three months from a 5.4 to a 7.8. I continued my juicing practice for another three months thinking that certain enzymes would ultimately kill the cancer cells in my prostate. My next PSA was 9.5 even though my other blood counts were perfect. It became clear to me that my remedies were not sufficient, and I needed to seek additional help.

To be perfectly clear, I strongly recommend a perpetual lifestyle of a nutritional diet. In today's society little interest is given to the nutritional value of foods. More emphasis is placed on additional chemicals to promote increased productivity and shelf preservation of food. With the increase of toxins in many areas of our environment, a deliberate lifestyle of nutritional habits is very important. However, I emphasize that a combination of nutritional eating habits and conventional medicine is the best way to combat prostate cancer.

Chapter 9

Hard Choices

Trust in the Lord with all thine heart; and lean not unto thine own understanding. In all thy ways acknowledge him, and he shall direct thy path.
Proverbs 3:5-6

After clearly establishing that prostate cancer was my problem, my urologist explained several treatment options to me. I guess you've gathered that I really admire my urologist. Even as I make observations such as I am about to make about the speed of his conversation, it is not intended to be destructive criticism. However, it was most difficult for me to digest the rapid explanation of treatment choices when I had not fully come to grips with my condition.

As I recall, he indicated that because of my age, he would recommend radical prostatectomy-- removal of the prostate gland and surrounding tissue. The operation would last up to four hours, require a hospital stay of three to seven days, and three to six weeks of recovery. The most likely candidates for this surgery are otherwise healthy men whose cancer has not spread outside of the prostate and who have a life expectancy of 10 years or more. He indicated that the side effects of surgery may include impotence and incontinence. I later learned that impotence is reported in 30-50 percent of patients in the first year after surgery.

He also mentioned radiation therapy. This treatment involved the use of X-rays to kill tumors and decrease their ability to grow. He specifically had reference to external beam therapy where patients receive X-ray treatments over six or seven weeks. The side effects of this treatment include temporary impotence and incontinence in 30-50 percent of patients. I learned of side effects such as: diarrhea, urinary retention and inflammation of the bladder, penis and scrotum. He stated that this is recommended for older men, those in poor health, or those with more advanced tumors. He quickly added that he did not recommend radiation as a treatment for me.

He also explained that hormonal therapy was a form of treatment, but is used mostly in men with advanced prostate cancer.

As my doctor hurriedly suggested that I have blood tests done to prepare for a radical prostatectomy, I immediately told him that I needed more time to consider my options.

I was fortunate to have a member from my congregation who was working in my urologist's office. He had a similar surgery and had almost no side effects. This parishioner, Bro. Ernest Bulluck, proved to be my greatest comforter in the midst of my struggle with the dilemma I faced. Ernest was a soft-spoken, very sincere and truthful friend. Clearly, God had wrought a miracle in his life through the surgery Dr. Whisnant had performed on him. The surgery was an overwhelming success. Ernest had no incontinence and had, by his own testimony, retained from 80-90% of his sexual function. No one could deny the outcome of his surgery was phenomenal, but not enough to convince me that I should choose surgery as my option.

I informed Dr. Whisnant that I needed more time to consider my options. The first thing I wanted to do was seek a second opinion. He went along with my decision, and agreed to arrange an appointment with another urologist. He also recommended several books that I could read to give me a greater understanding of the disease and the treatment options. He told me that this particular cancer was a slow-growing cancer and that many men 65 and older have nothing done but engage in a process of "waiting and watching." He strongly recommended that I choose some form of treatment because the research had shown that the disease grew faster in younger men than in older ones. He continued to express optimism that my disease could be successfully treated and encouraged me to have a positive attitude. His positive reinforcement played a great role in my recovery. However, I left his office with the intent of trying everything I could to prevent having surgery.

My urologist made an appointment with a doctor at another eastern North Carolina hospital for a second opinion. I was extremely disappointed at the outcome of that visit. Within two minutes after being seated in this doctor's office, after scanning over my report, he agreed that I had prostate cancer. Disappointedly, I asked him if he was going to examine me. He said it was not necessary, I had the disease, and that the only treatment he recommended was surgery; and if I didn't get the surgery, I would be dead before age 55. My righteous indignation reached the highest level it had in a long time. I was so disappointed in that visit that I never mentioned it to my urologist. Had it not been for the grace of God, this entire book would have taken a different form after that doctor's visit.

In seeking more information about treatment options, I contacted a variety of places which include:

American Cancer Society
American Prostate Society
Cancer Information Center
Howard University Cancer Center
Leo W. Jenkins Cancer Center
National Cancer Institute

Several months passed and I still had not made a decision on my method of treatment. I totally modified my eating habits, became a complete vegetarian, and kept a conscious check on my PSA, mostly through my family physician, Dr. Samuel Wesonga, whom I believe had several conferences with my urologist to express his concern about my lack of action in selecting a treatment.

Finally, my urologist, Dr. Joseph Whisnant, sent me a very direct letter expressing his grave concern over my "paralysis of analysis." He said I needed to do something right away because my PSA readings were increasing.

Both my family doctor and my urologist demonstrated a passionate concern for my well-being in light of my procrastination. I am sincerely grateful to have had them as my caretakers. It is very important to have trust and confidence in your doctor when faced with a serious disease like prostate cancer. My doctors seemed to be aware of my special needs and concerns. They were sensitive and caring. I felt that they not only sympathized with me, but empathized. However, I know I am not an easy patient because admittedly, preachers tend to advise others rather than listen to advice themselves.

Realizing that my major concerns about surgery were incontinence and impotence, my urologist arranged an appointment with Dr. Patrick Walsh at Johns Hopkins, who is noted for nerve-sparing surgery. This doctor's calendar was filled, and it would be months before he could do the surgery. However, he indicated that he could have a conference with me.

During my most recent visit with Dr. Whisnant, he too suggested that if I didn't do something it would result in my death. He seemed to agree that any medical treatment was better than nothing. In addition to discussing the option of external radiation, he introduced me to a treatment called brachytherapy or seeding. This process involved placing radioactive pellets, the size of a grain of rice, into cancerous regions for weeks or months.

Bingo!!!

My urologist scheduled an appointment for me to see Dr. Frederick Ellwanger, a radiologist at Nash General Hospital. Although I went to see him about external radiation, I could not get the internal seeding out of my mind. By the way, in case you're wondering, every time I visited the doctor, I had an unavoidable sidekick named Joyce, my African Queen. She seemed not to trust me to give her total information about my treatment plans, but rather preferred to hear it from the "horse's mouth."

As we sat patiently listening to the details of external radiation, I asked Dr. Ellwanger if he had heard of the seeding process. He smiled and said, "yes, I once worked with a group of urologists at the Urology Health Center in New Port Richey, Florida." He explained that they did a procedure called radiation seeding. We talked about a similar service in New York and also a doctor who formerly performed the procedure in Atlanta. Although he completed his orientation on external radiation, I left his office determined to continue the search for further information about the "seeding" process.

Chapter 10

Bingo!!! MY Treatment

. . .with his stripes we are healed.
Isaiah 53:5

Some days later, I recalled Dr. Ellwanger saying that he used to work with a urologist in New Port Richey, Florida. I contacted him to inquire about their services. I spoke to Dr. Jerrold Sharkey who informed me that he could see me in the next 2-3 weeks and told me to bring my charts from my local urologist. We made an appointment and I later flew into the airport in Tampa, Florida. I rented a car, and drove to New Port Richey, Florida, which is about 50 minutes away from Tampa. I had all kinds of mixed emotions because I'd never heard of a place called New Port Richey, Florida. I didn't know if

I would find a small, unsanitary office of a quack seeking to make a fast buck by making me a guinea pig. I also considered the possibility that I would simply just be turned down for other reasons.

After much searching, I found a large, modern complex full of some of the friendliest people I've ever met in my life. I felt cared for from the moment I talked to the receptionist to the time I sat down and talked to Dr. Sharkey and his assistants. He told me they were engaging in a procedure called radiation implant seeding. He asked me why didn't I want to take the radical prostatectomy. I explained to him my fears of side effects.

After asking a number of questions relating to my eligibility, he studied my charts closely. I was later shown a film which explained the seeding process. I also talked with the radiologist who explained more about the procedure. Then I was told that I would have to come back for a study and prep procedures which would amount to measuring me for the prostate seeds. Dr. Sharkey informed my local urologist to put me on Lupron shots for a period of three months to shrink the size of my prostate so it would not be necessary for them to cut any bones to get to my prostate area.

I drove back to the airport with a great sense of relief. I felt strongly that seeding was the way to go. I remember praising God for this revelation as I drove along Route 19 back to the airport.

For the next three months, once a month, I visited my urologist to receive an injection of Lupron Depot. Technically, Lupron is a chemical castration. It works by shutting down testosterone produced by the testicles, which causes a decrease in the amount of testosterone circulating in the body. Because it lowers testosterone, this drug helps relieve the pain, difficulty in urinating and other symptoms associated with prostate cancer.

If my doctor had asked me to take Lupron shots when I was first diagnosed with cancer, I probably would have been as pessimistic about the shots as I was the surgery. I experienced severe hot flashes and total impotence while on the shots. Some men experience a temporary increase in their urinary symptoms or pain during the initial weeks of Lupron treatment. The good news was it was only temporary.

In retrospect, I consider Lupron to be a wonder drug in the treatment of prostate cancer. Most doctors only prescribe Lupron for patients with advanced prostate cancer. As a layman, I wonder why it is not recommended to all prostate cancer patients while they are determining their choice of treatment. I am careful not to tell my doctor what to do; however, if my PSA ever starts to rise again, I trust he will immediately put me back on Lupron shots. I can deal with the hot flashes and the temporary impotence. The positive thing about Lupron is that it gave me a peace of mind that the testosterone was no longer fueling the growth of my cancer.

In early December 1996, approximately two weeks before I was to receive the radioactive seed implantation, I returned to New Port Richey, Florida to the diagnostic center. Dr. Sharkey and his staff carried me through a procedure he described as measurements for the radiation implants. I was given anesthesia while the medical staff measured me to determine the location and number of seeds I would receive. As I recall, I was given a preoperative ultrasound and CT scan, which was used to calculate the volume and position of my prostate. A computer was used to determine the amount of radiation needed and where the seeds should be placed. This was necessary to make sure that my treatment would be specifically designed for my problem. No two patients are given the same amount of seeds, nor are they necessarily placed in the same location in different patients.

Dr. Sharkey assured me that the planning and the execution of this procedure would be done with much care. Strangely enough, I never doubted him, although I had just met him. Guess who accompanied me on this trip--none other than the wonder lady herself, my wife, Joyce.

Each time I traveled to the diagnostic center I met other patients who had either received seeds and had come back for a follow-up or those like myself, who were about to undergo seed placement. They all seemed to feel very good about their prognosis and the care they were receiving from the Urology Health Center. I became more and more confident that the decision I was making was the right one and so did my faithful companion.

On December 18, 1996, I returned to the Urology Health Center in New Port Richey, Florida. My son, Rev. Timothy J. Walker, accompanied me on this trip because the anesthesia from my treatment and the catherization would necessitate stronger assistance than my wife was capable of rendering.

My first day at the Urology Health Center consisted of a series of tests and preparations for the procedure that would take place the following day. I was extremely impressed with the idea that instead of being confined to a hospital, I was able to stay at a nearby hotel before and after the procedure. At the conclusion of that day, I was given a bottle of colyte and told to take it and drink a gallon of water so that I would be cleaned out for the procedure.

The needles for the procedure were prepared the night before based upon the measurements taken earlier. I jokingly call this procedure "The Mustard Seed" Treatment, mainly because the radioactive seeds resemble mustard seeds. I remember the film I viewed during my first visit, which indicated that the implant seeds consist of a pointed stylet within a sleeve. When the stylet is taken out, the seeds are dropped into the hollow tube of the sleeve where they are deposited into the prostate gland.

December 19--**The Day**-- my son drove me to the diagnostic center around 8 o'clock that morning. The staff was well-organized. Every person I met from the receptionist to the attending medical staff in the recovery room were attentive to my every need. After undressing and carefully bagging my personal belongings, I was guided to a room where I was connected to an IV. My blood pressure was checked, and I was asked several questions to assure them I had followed the instructions given the day before.

I remember telling the anesthesiologist that I wasn't fond of lying still on my back, especially with my legs in stirrups. He assured me that as soon as I arrived in the operating room, they would apply the anesthesia and I would remember nothing. The next thing I remembered was being offered some orange juice and a Sara Lee muffin in the recovery room.

After being in the recovery room for approximately two hours, I was allowed to return to the hotel with my son. Although I was catheterized and extremely sedated, I remember rejoicing in my spirit that I had chosen this form of treatment.

The next day, we returned to the diagnostic center. I was sent to a neighboring medical facility and given a CT scan to assure that the seeds were properly placed. A few hours later, the catheter was removed, and I returned to the hotel to get a good night's sleep. Barring slight soreness, most of which resulted from the catherization, I felt great.

The doctor told me it would be necessary for me to refrain from holding babies and young children and being around pregnant women for the next six weeks. We also determined that it would be best if I slept in a separate bed from my wife for a few weeks. Those were the only restrictions of activities I was given, other than carefully judging the amount of weight I lifted. I felt very good about the treatment option I chose.

Dr. Sharkey asked Dr. Whisnant, my local urologist, to continue me on the Lupron shots at least two months after the seeding. I remember wondering why that was necessary. However, in retrospect, I believe the combination of prayer, the Lupron shots, the radiation seeds, and a nutritional diet caused me to receive the report you will read about in the chapter on my annual checkup.

Chapter 11

My Annual Checkup

Beloved, I wish above all things that thou mayest prosper and be in health, even as thy soul prospereth.
III John 2

The next year (from January 1997 until January 1998) was perhaps the longest year of my life. Having received the radiation seeds, I now had to wait for my annual checkup to see if the seeds were effective. It's hard to express the deep psychological trauma I experienced as I wondered about my prognosis.

Initially, I continued my research on prostate cancer as though I had not been treated. In retrospect, I guess I added to my dilemma by perpetually pondering over my findings. In fact, my family doctor replied, "You worry too much about what you're reading." He made this statement after hearing me complain of several symptoms that would indicate the cancer had advanced. Advanced prostate cancer means that the cancer has escaped from the prostate into other areas of the body. Clearly, my mind was playing tricks on me. I'd read that advanced prostate cancer is indicated by lower back pains, shoulder pains, hip and leg pains. I felt like I had all of the above. I reasoned that perhaps the seeds had not worked or had missed their target. I guess I thought the whole procedure was so strategic that it was highly possible that something had gone wrong. I thought I felt pain in every place the cancer could possibly spread, including my lymph nodes under my arms, neck and upper thigh. I spent an enormous amount of time thinking I had waited too long between the diagnosis of my condition and the treatment. To be honest, I was an emotional wreck. It is a wonder I was able to carry on my daily activities of providing pastoral care for others, while in such deep depression about my own health.

Little did my three grandchildren know that Pa Pa was as anxious to see Christmas 1997 as they were, but for a different reason. December 19 constituted one year from the time of my treatment, and I was scheduled to return to New Port Richey, Florida for my annual exam. I called the diagnostic center to schedule my appointment for the month of December. However, due to the Christmas holidays, I was scheduled for January 1998. That Christmas was one to remember.

Around January 12 my wife and I boarded a plane to Tampa, Florida. After arriving at the airport, we rented a car, as usual, and took a 45 minute drive to New Port Richey. I had mixed emotions about the extent I was willing to be examined because I had been told it would be intensive. However, Joyce encouraged me to be cooperative because, in her words, "You've come too far to start acting like a child now." Only a wife of 31 years can readjust one's ego with only eleven words. By the time we arrived at the diagnostic center, I was ready to submit to whatever they would subject me to.

We had a five-day reservation at the hotel because I had allowed four days for the examination and one day for rest and recuperation. On the first day, I was given an ultrasound. This imaging technique projects sound waves off the prostate and surrounding organs to create an image. Ultrasounds, in most cases, accurately identify the local spread of prostate cancer. While this was not the first ultrasound I'd ever experienced, it was my first experience with such a humorous and caring technician. I guess he could tell I was uptight, so his table-top manners (generally known as bedside manners) were superb. In spite of his intense effort to relax me with humor, my tension was increased when he indicated that there was a dark area that could be remnants of the cancer. So I wouldn't become too horrified, he hastened to say the dark spot could be the formation of the seeds in my prostate.

My fear that the cancer had spread to other areas of my body was at its greatest height as I left the ultrasound area. What happened next did not help calm my fears. I was given a digital rectal exam. The physician inserted a lubricated gloved finger into my rectum to feel for any hard spots he could detect. The physician informed me that he felt a hard spot in the same area the ultrasound had revealed. Further tests were to follow.

I was then sent to the hospital facility located within walking distance of the diagnostic center. In fact, I simply walked out the back door of the diagnostic center across the street to the hospital. My purpose was to take a bone scan to see if the cancer had spread to other parts of my body. I'm not sure whether the bone scan is a general procedure for annual examination, but given the fact I had complained of all of the symptoms that would indicate the spread of the cancer, Dr. Sharkey recommended a bone scan to be sure. After the bone scan, I went to the diagnostic center's lab to have my blood drawn and to give urine specimens.

The next day was a big day. I arrived at the diagnostic center around 8:00 a.m. It seemed as though history was repeating itself. I found myself going through the same general procedures I went through for the treatment. I checked in, undressed, received an IV, had my blood pressure checked, and was once again treated as though I were "king for the day." Only this time, I was being prepped for a 17-point biopsy. I am told it is the most thorough examination one can have to detect prostate cancer. Soon, I was in the recovery room again, but as inquisitive as I was about the outcome, no one told me anything. The suspense was killing me.

I returned to my hotel room and spent the evening relaxing and being encouraged by guess who? Yes, my African Queen was at her best, cheering me across the finish line, encouraging me to think positively and insisting that the doctor would have a good report for me. The night was long with anticipation of the doctor's report. Dr. Sharkey's assistant called the hotel the next day and set a time for me to come in and talk with him. I recall wondering in my mind, "talk with me." If we have to talk, there must be some concerns, I reasoned. I was thinking if the results were negative we wouldn't need to talk that much; he could just tell me they were negative, and I'll see you in another year. Surely, something was wrong!

Finally, the time arrived! This day reminded me of the day Joyce and I went in to see Dr. Whisnant, my local urologist, for the results of my first biopsy. The only difference was Joyce now was noticeably weaker as a result of her degenerating neurological condition. I knew the last thing she needed was more shocking news about my condition. I wondered if the results would be the same as that January day in 1996 when I was told the initial biopsy was positive--I had cancer. Much to my surprise our meeting with Dr. Sharkey was extremely brief and pleasant. He smiled and said, "The results of our tests were negative. We found no sign of cancer, and I'll see you next year this time." Needless to say, there was a hallelujah in my soul. I felt like running out of his office so the staff could not hear me shout for joy. The good news also seemed to have been medicine for Joyce as I sensed a sigh of relief from her.

Chapter 12

Taking Charge of the Temple

*What? Know ye not that your body is the temple
of the Holy Ghost which is in you, which ye
have of God, and ye are not your own?*
I Corinthians 6:19

There's an old adage that says, "An ounce
of prevention, is worth a pound of cure." If you
have prostate cancer or wish to avoid the disease,
you must take charge of your temple. While no
one is sure of the total cause of prostate cancer,
research has shown that smoking, diets high in
fats and salt, stress, and lack of rest greatly
contribute to the disease.

Nutrition and diet are important for the
prevention and treatment of prostate cancer. If
you have a proper diet, you will feel better and

have more energy. Your daily intake should include enough calories and protein to sustain your strength and rebuild normal tissues.

According to Prescription for Nutritional Healing, an anticancer diet is composed primarily of brown rice, fresh raw fruits and vegetables, fresh juices, legumes, raw nuts and seeds, and whole grains, and excludes alcohol, coffee, refined carbohydrates, and strong tea. A regular, daily intake of 50 milligrams of zinc and essential fatty acids in later life also may help prevent the development of problems.

Suggested Dietary Considerations

- Eat plenty of whole grains, raw nuts and seeds, and brown rice.

- Eat plenty of fresh fruits (especially apples, fresh cantaloupe, all kinds of berries, cherries, grapes, and plums).

- Include foods high in zinc, such as mushrooms, pumpkin seeds, seafood, spinach, and sunflower seeds.

- Limit your intake of dairy products.

- Use sesame, safflower or olive oil to obtain essential fatty acids.

- Minimize the intake of red meat.

- Eliminate diet drinks, alcoholic beverages, coffee, and all teas except caffeine-free herbal teas.

- Avoid: junk foods, processed refined foods, salt, saturated fats, sugar, and white flour.

Although the full impact of diet and exercise is not known, studies indicate that engaging in regular exercise might reduce the risk of prostate cancer.

Though I have been successfully treated for prostate cancer, I am extremely careful about how I treat my body, which is the temple of God. I am convinced that conscientious planning of my diet and health regiment will lessen the possibility of the cancer reoccurring. Remember the cliché, "You are what you eat" is worth considering when it comes to prostate health.

Chapter 13

Impotence???

...Wilt thou be made whole?
John 5:6

There is an almost unanimous concern among men about the loss of their sexual functions due to prostate cancer treatment. "An open confession is good for the soul" is a better way of putting it. I admit impotence was my foremost concern, especially as I struggled with the possibility of surgery. As I forestated, my good friend, Ernest Bulluck, reminded me that he retained at least 80-90% of his sexual function and experienced absolutely no incontinence after his surgery. Some men experience incontinence (which is uncontrollable leakage) as a result of surgery to the extent they have to wear bladder control pads. I was convinced that Ernest was an exception rather than a rule and I wasn't about to risk the loss of my sexual functions.

The longer I lived with the reality that I had prostate cancer and the more I read about how painful and deadly the disease could be, the less important sexual function became. Besides, I had seen several incidences where men had to have their testicles removed because the cancer had spread beyond the prostate.

As I saw my PSA rapidly increase from 5.4 to almost 10 points, the impotence concern moved from 100% to about 20%. In the large scheme of things, the effects of the Lupron shots were tolerable because, as I stated earlier, the side effects were temporary. As I learned about the seriousness of prostate cancer, my concern shifted from sex to survival. The psychological struggles of prostate cancer clearly eliminated concerns of impotence. However, after my annual checkup I noticed a restoration of sexual functions to almost a normal state. I contribute this not only to the type of treatment I selected, but the psychological release experienced after receiving a cancer-free report from Dr. Sharkey.

Problems with erection will vary based on the treatment choice, other physical problems and/or psychological problems. My research has shown that impotence is a common problem many men experience just with the announcement of prostate cancer. The psychological impact of such a disease is enough to impair *any* normal functions of the body, but especially sexual functions.

Fortunately, impotence is treatable. I would strongly urge my brother who may experience impotence as a result of prostate problems to seek professional help. Your urologist will help you determine whether your impotence is physical or psychological. Your physician will need a thorough medical history, lab tests, and a physical examination to determine the cause of your impotence.

There are a variety of options for treating impotence, let me mention a few.

Viagra
(The current Rolls Royce of impotence treatment)

a. What is Viagra? Viagra is a popular, new medication that is taken by mouth to restore erectile function in men with erectile dysfunction. It is the first of its kind. It works selectively on the penis. It is not a hormone or an aphrodisiac.

b. Is this drug safe? From the information I've been able to acquire, YES, it is. It has been tested in over 4,500 men over a three-year period. The incidence of adverse side effects causing patients to drop out of the studies was equal in patients taking placebo versus Viagra, 2.5%.

c. How does the pill work? Viagra works by increasing the smooth muscle relaxation in the penis. When an erection occurs, the smooth muscles in the penis and in the arteries of the penis must be relaxed. Viagra maximizes the relaxation increasing the efficiency of the erection. It is like stretching a rubber balloon before blowing it up to make it easier to inflate.

d. What are the side effects? Statistics reveal few side effects of using Viagra.

The national news media has clearly presented Viagra as a "cure-all" for men with impotence problems. However, if Viagra does not work for you, there are other treatments available such as:

1. Change of medication if your doctor senses your medication may be the problem.

2. Vacuum Erection Therapy - A chamber is placed over the penis and a vacuum is created that draws blood into the penis, causing an erection. The erection is maintained by a ring that is placed around the base of the penis.

3. Penile Self-Injection - This is a process of a brother giving himself a shot directly into his penis. This drug causes the blood vessels in the penis to relax, opening them up so blood can flow freely to the penile tissue. The penis generally becomes erect enough to enable you to have intercourse within 10-20 minutes.

4. Implant Surgery - If all else fails, you may choose the option of surgery. Implant surgery is a process of inserting a concealable, specially-fitted prosthesis along the upper side of the penis.

You will need to talk with your urologist concerning greater details of these methods of eliminating the problem of impotence. There are also organizations dedicated to helping men with impotence problems. For additional information contact:

Impotence Institute of America
2020 Pennsylvania Ave. NW, Suite 292
Washington, DC 20006
(800) 669-1603

The Impotence Institute of America is a non-profit organization that provides information and physician referrals.

I thought it was important that I include a chapter to speak to this sensitive issue because it is very grievous to me to realize how many men are neglecting proper diagnosis and treatment because of this grave concern.

Chapter 14

It Takes Faith

The just shall live by faith.
Romans 1:17

From one brother to another, or to the woman who is reading this book because of her concern for her man, let me declare that prostate cancer draws on your faith. In fact, were it not for a living faith in a living God, I would have given up amidst the journey. In my transparent moments, I realize I revealed times of fear and anxiety. True as that is, had I not had faith in God to balance the human frailty, I would have truly lost my mind. The belief of my support group, drum-majored by my wife, Joyce, and a broad base of support from family and friends helped to undergird my own faith.

God has a way of giving you what you need when you need it. A few days after being diagnosed with prostate cancer, I had a revival at our church. Dr. H. Beecher Hicks, Pastor of the Metropolitan Baptist Church of Washington, DC and the author of the best-seller book "Preaching Through A Storm," was our evangelist. I'm not sure of the total effect the revival had on my congregation, but I do know, each night he preached made my faith in God a little bit tighter and my future much brighter. I did not mention my condition to Dr. Hicks, but I am truly indebted to him for allowing God to use him to minister to my congregation and me. Faith truly comes by hearing, and hearing by the Word of God.

While this book is not intended to be a book of sermons or an effort to convert anyone to my belief, I do not apologize for boldly declaring that faith in God's Word will work in any situation. That is why I begin each chapter with a scripture.

I believe three elements are necessary to survive prostate cancer. III John 2 says, "Beloved I wish above all things that thou may prosper and be in health even as your soul prosper." The three elements are (1) a strong faith and devotion to God, (2) a thorough knowledge of your body functions and how good nutrition, rest, and exercise are foundational for good health, and (3) a willingness to search out treatment options, seek second opinions, join support groups, and realize that even medical science is a manifestation of God's power.

I've talked with many men who are faced with the problem of prostate cancer. Some are being treated for a cancer that is still contained within the prostate. Others are faced with the challenge of day-by-day survival as they face the awesome reality that the cancer has spread beyond the prostate. I have even shared my experience with groups of men within my own congregation and throughout the community. On more than one occasion, men who were present during my lectures have gone to the doctor and were examined only to find that they too had prostate cancer. My advice to them was to "lift up their eyes unto the hills from whence comes their help, for our help comes from the Lord."

The greatest testimony of faith I've witnessed is that of a college professor who once taught at Shaw University, my alma mater. He was diagnosed with prostate cancer over 25 years ago, discovered by a digital rectal exam. Twenty-five years ago PSAs were not used to detect prostate cancer. Each year he received a digital rectal exam to determine the health of his prostate, but nothing was found. About four years ago he suffered a light heart attack which necessitated hospitalization. While in the hospital, the doctor suggested he have a PSA test. He agreed, but unfortunately the PSA reading was above 66 points. The cancer had escaped the prostate. He later had his testicles removed to slow down the growth of the cancer because as I forestated, prostate cancer grows from testosterone, which is like kerosene on a fire. I mention him because he embodies the greatest demonstration of faith in the midst of advanced prostate cancer I have ever witnessed. He openly and freely discusses his condition with survivor groups through local chapters of the American Cancer Society. He boldly declares that through faith in God, he is surviving one day at a time. In fact, each time I see him he asks for another copy of my record of the same title because he stated he had literally worn the other copy out. I trust I can encourage others to have faith like him.

Coming from a Christian home, prayer has always been a focal point for me. We were always taught to say our prayers; however, prostate cancer will stop you from just saying prayers and start you really praying prayers. There is a difference. Remember, "the victory that overcomes the world is our faith." Sometimes I wonder why God allowed me to experience this problem, but when I consider the many men I've already shared my story with and those who will be instructed by this book, I understand that God has a purpose that must be received by faith. Never give up on your faith in God regardless of the forecast. This is my message to men and women everywhere, "Your faith in God will see you through."

Chapter 15

Confirmation of Facts

Wisdom is the principal thing; therefore get wisdom: and with all thy getting get understanding.
Proverbs 4:7

The word confirmation is synonymous with corroboration, documentation, authentication, and verification. That is what this book is all about--a documentation from my perspective. The last thing we need to do concerning prostate cancer, or any other disease, is to try to parade ourselves as being original. The truth of the matter is that "facts are facts." The most interesting part of the research in writing this book is the repetition of the materials I found. Therefore, the aim of this book is not to be original, but to be unique in my own way and reach an audience that maybe others have not reached.

To illustrate the similarities of the problem, a friend of mine from the Atlanta area sent me an article from The Atlanta Journal/The Atlanta Constitution dated Sunday, September 2, 1997. This article reaffirms the same concerns and issues I see voiced over and over again. Consider the following scenario:

Diagnosis of Prostate Cancer
Treatment Recommendation
Contemplation of Treatment Methods
Decision
Treatment

Let's consider each step in the above scenario:

<u>Diagnosis of Prostate Cancer</u>. The diagnosis of prostate cancer may come as a result of a routine physical examination or an examination requested as the result of problems noted by the patient. In either case, the news is a staggering announcement.

Questions and confusion seem to plague the minds of men confronted with this crisis. What? Why? How? When? What is this cancer that's invaded my body? Why is this happening? and Why is it happening to me? How could this happen? When did this happen? Study after study, along with my personal experiences, support the state of disequilibrium in which a man diagnosed with prostate cancer finds himself.

Treatment Recommendation. According to Dr. Patrick Walsh, urologist-in-chief at Johns Hopkins Hospital in Baltimore and a top authority in the field, there is no simple, uniform answer on how to treat prostate cancer. He encourages men to seek several doctors' opinions, read about the disease, and take the advice of the physician they trust most.

John Henkel, staff writer for FDA Consumer, says that the recommended choice of treatment depends on which specialist the patient consults. Urologists tend to recommend surgery while oncologists generally advise radiation therapy.

Repeatedly, my research indicates that there is a widespread recommendation for surgical removal of the prostate (prostatectomy) when the diagnosis is confined to the prostate. This is the same recommendation that was given to Hosea Williams who was described in the Atlanta newspaper article and to me.

Contemplation of Treatment Methods by Patient. Once the unsettling news starts to sink in as truth, the struggle over treatment methods begins. Surgery? Radiation? Hormone Therapy? Watchful Waiting? It is important to seek information in an effort to make the right decision. Quality of life after treatment is a key issue for most men in determining the method of treatment.

Decision. When selecting an appropriate treatment, many factors must be considered carefully. What are the pros and cons? What are the benefits and complications? What are the risks? The decision not only affects the cancer patient, but all those who play a major role in the patient's life. It is extremely important that the patient makes an informed decision.

Treatment. Once a treatment method has been chosen, the patient must select a treatment facility and move forward with confidence in the decision he has made.

For men who are potential targets of this disease, it is important that you avail yourselves to all information available concerning your health. Don't sit idly by the sidelines and fail to take an active role in your own health. Be informed! Know the facts about prostate cancer.

What are the facts? Let's examine a few of them to see.

- One of every 10 American men will develop prostate cancer at some time in his life.

- Prostate cancer is the most common cause of cancer in men and the second leading cause of cancer deaths in men.

- Prostate cancer is usually curable when caught and treated before it spreads.

- Early prostate cancer causes no symptoms.

- The digital rectal examination is a simple office procedure which allows your doctor to detect many prostate cancers before symptoms develop.

- In 1997, 41,800 American men died and another 209,000 were diagnosed with prostate cancer.

- African Americans have the highest risk of developing prostate cancer.

- Having a father or brother with prostate cancer greatly increases a man's likelihood of developing the disease.

- Diets high in fat may contribute to prostate cancer.

"Wisdom is the principal thing; therefore get wisdom: and with all thy getting get understanding."

Chapter 16

The Wife's Dilemma
by
Mrs. Joyce Walker

For the husband is the head of the wife, even as Christ is the head of the church...
Ephesians 5:23

It's the happiest day of your life. For as long as you can remember, this is the day you've dreamed about. Even as a child, so many of the play activities were directed to this very day--the day you would marry the man of your dreams. And, of course, live happily ever after. For on that wedding day, all the dreams for a beautiful future are ahead.

Yet, those marriage vows alert you that there may be impending problems lying ahead. For better or worse? In sickness or in health?

Till death we do part? We all agree, but never really believe that serious sickness will come our way. Then **B - O - O - O - M!!!**

The worst!

The sickness!!

And maybe even the death!!!

All these things are confronting you as you are faced with the disturbing news that your husband has prostate cancer. Almost instantly, a world of dreams are shattered. Fear and anxiety are so overwhelming. You fear losing someone you love so much. Fear of the unknown somehow becomes your dominant emotion.

In the midst of all you're feeling, you realize more than anything else that your husband is experiencing your fears and some additional ones of his own. Without a doubt, you must be strong. After all, he needs you more than ever.

What Can You Do For Your Husband?

Support Your Husband

As your husband is dealing with the disease that has stricken his body, you must realize it is **his** body. Though the decision will impact you both and you should discuss treatment methods, ultimately, the decision is his.

Accompany Him To His Doctor's Visits

No matter how masculine or "macho" your husband may be, the news of prostate cancer has shaken his world at the very core. He needs your emotional support, but he also needs your physical support. Be there for him and with him whenever you can.

Appoint Yourself as His Personal Research Assistant

One of the first things your husband will need to do is gather all the information he can on prostate cancer and treatment methods. Accompany him to the library and bookstores. Help him surf the internet. Explore every possible treatment method available. Locate treatment centers and gather information on them. Encourage him to talk with other prostate cancer survivors. Do whatever you can to insure that your husband's decision is an informed one. Your future together depends upon it.

Give Him Space

Your initial response may be to shower him with sympathetic expressions or insist that he should talk about what he's feeling. Sounds good! But remember this is a devastating announcement. Although, as a woman, this may be exactly what you need to do when confronted with adverse conditions or news in your life, your husband may be quite the opposite. He may need to find his own time and his own space. When he's ready, he'll talk about it. Just remember not to rush him. When he's ready, he'll open up and share his feelings with you.

Validate His Masculinity

Depending on the stage of his cancer, your husband may not be able to function in his normal roles. He may not be able to provide the financial support he once did. He may not have the physical strength to carry on his normal daily activities. His treatment choice may have left him impotent or incontinent. It is imperative that you show concern for his physical as well as emotional well-being. Assure him that your life is not contingent upon his physical characteristics or his being able to perform certain physical functions. The physical closeness that you share with him, such as hugging, cuddling and kissing will help reassure him that he is still very desirable to you.

Love Him

Nothing can mean more to your husband at this time than your unconditional love. With the core of his manhood being challenged, it is imperative that he understand that you love everything about him. If you haven't done so lately, you may want to "spell out" all the things you love about him. Reassure him of your love, but don't overdo it to the point of becoming superfluous.

What Can You Do For You?

Face Your Fears

Although your whole world may seem to be caving in around you, remember that your husband's fears are probably far greater than yours. For him, this problem attacks the very essence of his manhood. You must learn to deal with your fears by facing each one of them head-on. There's an old cliché that says, "there's nothing to fear, but fear itself." If your fears are compounded because you don't know what to expect from this disease, then read and learn all you can about it. If you fear the complications that result from treatment, read and learn all you can about the various methods of treatment. If you fear the loss of intimacy in your relationship because of impotence, remember that sex is only one aspect of intimacy. If your greatest fear is that you will lose your spouse to this dreadful disease, remember that "all sickness is not unto death." Review the statistics on cures and maintain a positive attitude.

Find Strength Through Others

Remember, no man or woman is an island, and whatever you're feeling or going through is not a situation unique to only you. You may find it very comforting to hear how other wives are dealing with this problem. Talking with a minister or counselor may be of some help to you in dealing with this difficult issue. You may even be surprised to know that you can be a source of strength, comfort and encouragement to other women experiencing the same thing.

Pray

I would certainly be remiss if I failed to mention the power of prayer in dealing with prostate cancer or any problem. This is definitely a time to draw closer to a Heavenly Father who sees all, knows all, and has all power. He healed the sick and raised the dead nearly 2,000 years ago. He will do no less now. For "Jesus Christ is the same yesterday, today, and forever."

Needless to say, a deep spiritual relationship will be your greatest source of strength in a time like this. Although you may have family and friends who wish to help, learn to look to God, who invites us to cast all our cares upon him because he cares for us. Learn to lean on and trust in God and come to know the joy of serving him--for the joy of the Lord is your strength. Be encouraged, my sister.

Prostate Cancer Overshadows Other Problems

The dilemma of my husband's prostate cancer was compounded by my own physical condition. We were ambushed by the unexpected in 1988 when I was diagnosed with oligoponto-cerrebullar atrophy (a shrinkage of the cerebella of the brain), a hereditary disease that had taken the life of my father, my only brother at age 33, and several of my uncles. I said the unexpected because until I was diagnosed, we had no record of a female having this disease. Clearly, we thought as awful as the disease is, it only affected the males of our family. How wrong we were.

In addition, my mother, who seemed to have been a tower of strength, especially in dealing with this degenerating disease that claimed one family member after another, died in 1993. Lorenzo, my husband's middle name (a name exclusively reserved for use by his mother, his sister, and me), has demonstrated an unwavering love for me. I felt so secure in the fact that if God chose not to heal me, Lorenzo would be there for me as the disease progressed. Now it appeared that both of us may find ourselves in a position of needing home health care at best, and I feared to think of the worst. I spent many sleepless nights pondering over our future because he had always been a great protector and provider for our family. The real dilemma for me was to wonder what was going on in his mind as he experienced the physical and psychological stress of his illness. Suddenly, I realized that my concern for my own physical condition had diminished as I clinged closer to him in an effort to bring comfort.

Hold On! Help Is On The Way!

In January 1998, as we traveled to New Port Richey, Florida, for my husband's first annual check-up, I prayed without ceasing for good results. It is amazing how circumstances can change your prayer priorities. My usual prayer when I know we are going to travel by air is that the Lord will keep the pilot alert and the plane in the air. As we arrived at the Tampa airport and rented a car to take a 45 minute drive to New Port Richey, there was a strange silence that came over me. I was obsessed with perpetual prayer and meditation for good news of healing for the most important man in my life, with the exception of Jesus Christ.

Words cannot express the joy I felt when Dr. Sharkey told Lorenzo his tests were negative and that he had found no cancer whatsoever. Almost three years earlier I had sat with my husband to receive the shocking news that he had prostate cancer. That day I seemed to have entered into a great wilderness of fear, doubt, frustration, and yes, even anger. But with Dr. Sharkey's announcement, my whole world was illuminated with the glory of God. I knew the Lord had wrought another miracle. The Lord had used my worst nightmare to help me endure my own condition. In fact, I shared this revelation with my husband one day as we rode along through the countryside. "Lorenzo, as we wait on my healing I truly praise God for his loving kindness. I understand now as never before what God must be doing as he healed your body and I am still diseased." Lorenzo seemed to have been puzzled by my statement and asked, "Honey, what do you mean?" I said, "God has healed your body so that you can be here for me when I am not able to take care of myself." Lorenzo later mentioned in a sermon the profoundness of my statement and expressed to me a similar revelation. He said, "I've always loved you and from the day we married I've resolved to love you as I love my own body. My sickness and deliverance simply further solidify my commitment to be there for you regardless of what the future holds." Wives, I guess in a nutshell, I am saying, keep the lines of communication open and always remember what my husband reminded me of almost every day of our marriage, "we must take life's problems and make them life's projects."

Chapter 17

Comments From The Author's Children

Children are an heritage of the Lord... Happy is the man that hath his quiver full of them...
Psalm 127:3-5

Not Cancer--Not My Daddy!

Written by author's daughter, Teresa Walker-Mason, Esq.

On an August Evening in 1996, my sister-in-law was speaking to my mother and me about someone close to her who was dying of AIDS. I remember thinking, "This is the closest that I had ever come to actually knowing someone who is dying of that dreadful disease." At that moment, I silently thanked God for the blessing of good health. Soon, my sister-in--law left and I continued rolling my mother's hair for bed, as I

149

did most nights. A few moments later, my mother told me what I considered to be the most devastating news of my entire life.

"Your father has a serious disease," she said.

I was COMPLETELY SILENT for about 45 seconds. What disease? I asked. I could hardly breathe.

Cancer, she replied in his "prostrate." I immediately knew that she was referring to the prostate, an organ that is somehow related to a man's reproductive system.

You mean his prostate?, I replied.

Yes, he didn't want me to tell you because he knew you were studying for the bar exam.

Immediately, I retreated to my room and sobbed. As I sought to grasp the inconceivable notion that my daddy had cancer, I reflected on the recent changes in his lifestyle. For several months, Dad had drastically changed his eating habits. He was investing hundreds of dollars a month on natural and herbal remedies. He had purchased a top-notched juicer to liquefy vegetables and fruit such as: Carrots, Broccoli, Mustard Greens, Turnips, Watercress, Beets, Papaya, all of which was usually organic. He would always mix several of these vegetables together. The final product was a horrific-looking concoction that he would drink without even a quiver. He had lost over fifty pounds, mainly because his diet consisted only of those concoctions, beans, herbs, distilled water and grape juice. He would go to the local YMCA and spend hours in the sauna, "sweating out the toxins," he would say.

Having witnessed all of this, I hadn't a clue that he was ill. He seemed to have more energy than ever before, his skin looked as smooth as silk; he was preaching every Sunday at church as if all was well.

My daddy has always said, "We must take life's problems and make them life's projects." This man has more fight and tenacity than three or more Olympiads put together. He is always dreaming, always striving to make those dreams real, and unlike most people, always accomplishing them. After all is said and done, he gives the glory to God.

That August night, I sat up, wiped my tears, and realized that my dad had been fighting a battle. At that moment, I committed myself to helping him beat this disease. A couple days later, I told him that I knew what he was doing and vowed to help him get through this. Even then, dad expressed his desire to write a book about his healing of prostate cancer. This was before he had received any medical treatment for his condition. His faith and optimistic attitude made me feel crazy for having cried when I heard the news.

I later discovered that everyone else in the family knew about dad's condition long before I did. I initially resented that I was not let in on something so important. Everyone in the family knew that I felt I had discovered the phrase, "daddy's girl." Even today, my husband feels that he plays second fiddle to my dad. Although I had been consumed with studying for the Georgia Bar Examination that summer, I felt betrayed that everyone had kept me in the dark.

In retrospect, I appreciate my dad's decision to wait on telling me. I understand now that dad was sincerely dealing with a "secret storm." Knowing him like I do, I am sure that he would rather to have been told of his condition when he was alone. I am thankful, however, that my mom was there to lend her support. I appreciate the fact that he needed time to sort through the many personal alternatives that confronted him. Most importantly, he needed time to focus on God and seek the direction that He wanted him to move toward.

I attribute dad's healing of prostate cancer to the magnificent power of God. I also believe that my dad's healing is partly due to his undying determination to beat this disease through research and by taking charge of his "temple."

As I write this brief chapter, I have a great sense of pride. I am proud that Dad not only is continuing to maintain optimum health; he is writing his book to encourage other men to become survivors of prostate cancer.

Thanks, Dad, for allowing others to learn from your experience. More importantly, Dad, thanks for SURVIVING.

Like Father, Like Son

Written by author's son, Rev. Timothy J. Walker

There's a popular saying "like father, like son." I've always appreciated that cliché until the day I heard the dreadful announcement that my father had prostate cancer. Daddy knows I'm not saying this to disassociate myself with him by any stretch of the imagination, but his own research has shown that I have reason to be concerned not only about myself but about my son. Studies have shown prostate cancer to be hereditary. Therefore, I would advise all readers who have a family history of prostate cancer to take special steps to be sure that you are checked by your urologist on a regular basis.

I am simply ecstatic about the hard work my father has done on this book. The time, labor, research and meditation he has devoted to this project will probably never be known. Daddy has always been determined to take life's problems and make them life's projects, but this time he has outdone himself. Millions could be saved from the dreadful disease of prostate cancer as a result of this book. The knowledge I have acquired by assisting in the proofreading of this book has both raised and calmed fears in me concerning this dreadful disease. I am sure my son and I are equipped with the knowledge we need to protect ourselves from undetected prostate problems.

As a personal note to you, Daddy, please be assured that we will continue to support you and Mama as you seek to serve this generation. I am sure you will be called upon to speak to many support groups and even testify before legislative bodies about your findings. Please know that you have my support as you journey on this benevolent mission.

Chapter 18

Conclusion

Let us hear the conclusion of the whole matter...
Ecclesiastes 12:13

I trust the information contained in this book will be a great help to you and your loved ones. I have tried to speak from my heart through my own personal experiences from one brother to another. I especially thank the women who love their men enough to take the time to read this book written in layman's terms. I am sure it has equipped you with the necessary information to love your man into action that may save his life.

My brother, I've shared extensively about a walnut-sized member of your body which if kept healthy will aid the total body in a very meaningful and pleasurable way. I shall forever be affected by not only my bout with prostate cancer, but the knowledge of the millions whose lives are touched daily by this devastating disease. Yes, we know of millions, but many others are caught up in their own secret storms after being diagnosed with this dreadful disease. My prayer is that as a result of this book and efforts of great organizations such as the **National Prostate Cancer Coalition, American Cancer Society,** etc. and other individuals, more men will visit their urologists for regular checkups. The more early detections, the more lives will be saved. But, my brother, the disease must not only be detected early, but treated early and decisively.

I would be remiss if I did not express my deep concern for those who are unable to receive proper diagnosis and treatment due to their economic status. Clearly, the health delivery system in our country has much to be desired when it comes to meeting the needs of some low to moderate income citizens. I applaud the National Prostate Cancer Coalition and other organizations for their efforts to get more funding for the research of prostate cancer, and I hope that some organization or individual will champion more causes to see that everyone who needs and desires medical treatment will be afforded the opportunity to receive it.

The Big "C" is not a common cold or something to wink at. It is an issue of life and death and too often results in the latter. A special note to African American men--we are faced with an epidemic of prostate cancer. We can ill-afford to get bogged down in the "paralysis of analysis." I applaud the special efforts of the 100 Black Men working in concert with other groups to bring a greater focus on the seriousness of this problem especially among African American men. We can improve this statistic, but we must not forget that while some argue that we are not our brother's keeper, we are our brother's brother.

Don't play around with this dreadful disease. While I know the importance of nutritional diets, I do not recommend that anyone ignore the medical advances that have been made and try to fix this problem through vitamins and herbs alone. Make the hard choices quickly. Someone once told me, "if you study long, you study wrong." There's a medical treatment out there for you--Go for it.

In the words of the Apostle Paul in Ephesians 6:10 "Finally, my brethren, be strong in the Lord, and in the power of his might."

With much love and concern,

Your Brother, Thomas L. Walker

Unless otherwise noted, all Scripture quotations are from the King James Version.

Appendix A

National, State, and Local
Plan of Action

If continued progress is to be made in the fight against prostate cancer, there must be an aggressive local, state, and national plan of action. According to CaP CURE, the Association for the Cure of Cancer of the Prostate, "9.7 million American men have prostate cancer, and most don't even know it."

In my research, I have discovered several national initiatives with state and local components. We need not attempt to "re-invent the wheel." We must seek to develop coordinated efforts against this terrible disease.

I will not list the full details of all the action plans I discovered in my research. However, the following are some organizations that are making a tremendous impact in this important fight:

The National Prostate Cancer Coalition

NPCC's 1998 Action Plan is an aggressive, but workable, strategy that focuses on four important goals:

*   **Mobilizing and building grassroots constituency around the country into a major force for action and change;**

*   **Continuing to be a key player in the Halls of Congress, throughout Washington, DC, and in the media in the fight to increase federal funding for prostate cancer research;**

*   **Continuing important efforts to actively educate the public on prostate cancer and finding a cure, and broadening the base of**

support for prostate cancer research
funding; and

* Taking advantage of the election season to
  raise the issue of prostate cancer around the
  nation.

The NPCC has an excellent record of progress. Less than two years ago, NPCC was still an idea and a commitment by a group of individuals with a vision. Today, that vision is a reality and NPCC is poised to work with patients, survivors, families, doctors, researchers and coalition allies on their mutual mission to insist that when it comes to prostate cancer, our nation's officials take notice and take action.

NPCC Chairman, Bob Samuels, testified the fall of 1997 before the President's Panel and outlined priority areas for action on prostate cancer that he recommended be brought to the attention of the President.

In October—the NPCC Board adopted a budget of $1.6 million for 1998 to implement their aggressive advocacy program. For a complete copy of their action plan, contact:

Jay H. Hedlund, President and CEO
1156 15th Street, NW, Suite 905
Washington, DC 20005
Tel: (202) 463-9455

The American Cancer Society
Centers for Disease Control and Prevention
National Cancer Institute

The American Cancer Society, CDC (Centers for Disease Control and Prevention), and the National Cancer Institute sponsored A Leadership Conference on "Prostate Cancer in the African-American Community: An Agenda for Action," in Houston, Texas November 20-22, 1997. During the conference, they developed a Prostate Cancer National Blueprint for Action.

The Leadership Conference outlined action steps to be undertaken in the following areas:

* **Research in Basic and Behavioral Science**
* **Health Promotion and Education Based on Science**
* **Education and Support for Patients**
* **Public Policy**

It was a great leadership conference, and the plan of action is both aggressive and achievable. To receive a copy of the Prostate Cancer National Blueprint for Action, you may contact:

American Cancer Society
1599 Clifton Road, N.E.
Atlanta, Georgia 30329
Tel: (800) ACS-2345

100 Black Men of America

This is an organization working in conjunction with the American Cancer Society and other cancer associations and organizations in the fight against prostate cancer, especially in African American men.

Florida Prostate Cancer Action Network

The Florida Prostate Cancer Action Network held a strategy meeting December 13, 1997. The meeting was coordinated by one I refer to as "The General" in the fight against prostate cancer, Bob Samuels. The purpose of the meeting was to form a state-wide action plan on. . .

Research Funding
Medical Issues
Advocacy

Clearly, Bob Samuels is an example of the kind of person needed in every town, city, county, and state in our nation. FPCAN developed a form that I would recommend to be used in all local communities. The form is designed to enlist volunteers to join in the frontline fight against prostate cancer. I would also highly recommend that you request a copy of the Committee Hearing Bill; Health Care Services, Bill No. PCS/HB 1213. This is an excellent bill that was presented to the Florida House of Representatives and could be modified for local use. For more information, contact:

> Bob Samuels, Chairman
> Board of Directors
> National Prostate Cancer Coalition
> 8509 Woodwick Court
> Tampa, Florida 33615
> Tel: (813) 886-2171

There are many other effective national efforts in the fight against prostate cancer, such as:

> American Foundation for Urologic Disease
> 300 West Pratt Street, Suite 401
> Baltimore, MD 21201-2463
> Tel: (800) 242-2383

Cancer Information Service (CIS)
National Cancer Institute (NCI)
9000 Rockville Pike
Bethesda, MD 20892
Tel: (800) 4-CANCER

The Matthews Foundation For Prostate
   Cancer Research
1010 Hurley Way, Suite 195
Sacramento, CA 95825
Tel: (800) 234-6284

US TOO!
Prostate Cancer Survivor Support Groups
930 North York Road, Suite 50
Hinsdale, Illinois 60521-2993

I am sure I have not included all of the cancer-fighting agencies in the above list. However, I believe a knowledge of some of the resource groups available will help you develop your local action plan.

There are also many individual efforts. Wenda Royster is to be commended for her outstanding work and fight against cancer through her radio talk program in Baltimore, Maryland and Washington, DC. Wenda stresses the importance of good health and fitness. She can be heard on WOL 1450 AM in Washington and on 1010 AM in Baltimore.

Steps For Developing Your Local Plan of Action

Before you formulate the local plan, you should know the local statistics pertaining to prostate cancer. Our city, Rocky Mount, North Carolina, is uniquely located in two counties, Nash and Edgecombe.

Our Local Statistics Pertaining to Prostate Cancer

Here are some figures pertaining to prostate cancer in Nash and Edgecombe Counties provided by Area L AHEC:

- From 1991-1993, the total number of reported cases for Nash County: 160

- From 1991-1993, the total number of reported cases for Edgecombe County: 104

- There is a prostate cancer rate for Nash County of 143 cases/100,000 population.

- The rate for Edgecombe County is 141 cases/100,000 population.

- In Nash County, from 1991-95, there were 38 deaths among men aged 65-84 and 62 deaths over all age groups. The death rate for prostate cancer in Nash County for those years was 208/100,000 population in the 65-84 year age group and 21/100,000 population over all.

- The death rate for white males was 14.9/100,000 population and for all minorities it was 39.9/100,000 population.

- In Nash and Edgecombe Counties, this disease ranks among the top ten causes of death.

According to the American Cancer Society: Facts and Figures - 1998, North Carolina ranks in the top ten in prostate cancer cases.   It is estimated that there will be 5,600 incidences and 1,200 deaths in 1998.

Our Local Action Plan

- Identify as many prostate cancer support groups, survivors, and family members as possible.

- Organize a community task force aimed at promoting community awareness of prostate cancer.

- Develop strategies for expanding public awareness of prostate cancer, especially in the rural areas.

- Work collaboratively with county Health Departments, Area L AHEC, Region L, and other agencies to assist in promoting prostate cancer awareness.

- Appoint a committee to develop a proposed legislative action to be submitted to the NC House of Representatives, similar to House Bill 1213, which was developed by the Florida

Prostate Cancer Network, under the leadership of Bob Samuels.

- Appoint special committees to oversee coordination of our local efforts with state and national initiatives, such as a special committee to coordinate the signing and collection of "Petitions to the President of the United States and the Members of the United States Congress," developed by NPCC. A form is in the back of this book.

We can win this battle against this dreadful disease by faith in God and working with one another. Remember, you may be the person God has placed on planet Earth at this particular moment to make a difference in your own community in this important effort.

Appendix B

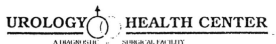

UROLOGY HEALTH CENTER

A DIAGNOSTIC & SURGICAL FACILITY

3499 MEADOW LANE, NEW PORT RICHEY, FL 34652, PHONE (813) 842-9441, FAX (813) 848-7230

Stanley D. Chovnick, M.D., F.A.C.S.
DIPLOMATE AMERICAN BOARD OF UROLOGY

Raymond J. Behar, M.D., F.A.C.S.
DIPLOMATE AMERICAN BOARD OF UROLOGY

Jerrold Sharkey, M.D., F.A.C.S.
DIPLOMATE AMERICAN BOARD OF UROLOGY

Ramon Perez, M.D., F.A.C.S.
DIPLOMATE AMERICAN BOARD OF UROLOGY

Juan N. Obregon, M.D., F.A.C.S.
DIPLOMATE AMERICAN BOARD OF UROLOGY

Richard L. Rabinowitz, M.D.

May 5, 1998

Reverend Thomas L. Walker
1026 Sycamore Street
Rocky Mount, North Carolina 27801

Dear Reverend Walker:

The diagnosis of prostate cancer is a life changing event for any
man with this problem. Reverend Walker has done an outstanding
job in enumerating the emotional and physical problems of the
disease. He has also taken you step-by-step through the process
and diagnosis to getting various opinions on treatment
alternatives to making the decision for his treatment.

A word of caution, there is no one treatment that is appropriate
for all patients with prostate cancer. Radical surgery is
appropriate for some, radiation therapy is appropriate for some,
seed implantation is appropriate for some, hormonal treatments
are appropriate for some and combinations of all of these
treatments are appropriate for some patients. One must have a
doctor or doctors that are well-versed in all these aspects of
treatment to help guide a patient through the decision making
process without bias. The most important point, I think, of this
book that is a common theme on all pages is **prevention, early
diagnosis, routine yearly exams.** We cure patients with prostate
cancer, but we only cure those patients who are found early
without symptoms, preferably on the basis of an abnormal PSA or
rectal examination and with a low volume of cancer. When it is
found when unsuspected or not on the basis of a yearly follow up,
the cancer is often very difficult to treat. The major lesson of
the book is what Reverend Walker speaks over and over and over
again about - don't be ashamed to go get a checkup.

Sincerely,

Jerrold Sharkey, M.D., F.A.C.S.

173

Prostate cancer is the number one cancer present in men. Although this year more men will be diagnosed with a new lung cancer, there will be almost <u>four</u> times as many men living with prostate cancer. African American men have the highest rate of prostate cancer in our country and in the world . I have read with rapt interest Reverend Walkers journey through the maze of diagnosis and treatment of his Prostate cancer. This narrative is particularly compelling to me as his physician as I was intricately involved with him in the decision making process. As a Urologist dealing with this tumor on a daily basis, Reverend Walkers' struggle to gain information and to make a treatment decision that was right for him has given me a special insight into the depths of soul searching required for any man to make this difficult decision.

He now has done a very special thing in writing this book and attempting to make more men aware of this insidious disease and the opportunity present for screening men for early diagnosis and treatment that can result in cure. I have no doubt that this book will save men's lives. I appreciate his attention to the medical detail and the obvious time and diligence required for a laymen to compile this excellent volume. I can only hope with Reverend Walker that more men, particularly African American men, will avail themselves of the information and insight in this book.

Joseph D Whisnant jr

Joseph D. Whisnant, Jr. M.D.

Appendix B

BOICE·WILLIS CLINIC

Rocky Mount, North Carolina

May 13, 1998

Rev. Thomas L. Walker
1026 Sycamore Street
Rocky Mount, North Carolina 27804

Chart#: 161

Dear Rev. Walker:

It was a privilege to be allowed to read the draft for your book on prostate cancer and your personal experience with it.

As I told you during my brief discussion in the hospital, your talent is with the spoken and written Word and is far better talent than any I have been given. I think your work is excellent and I enjoyed reading it personally. I was also struck by your devotion to your wife and also her chapter in the book.

At any rate, let me be the first one to buy your book once it is published.

Sincerely,

BOICE-WILLIS CLINIC, P.A.

Stuart K. Todd, M.D.

SKT:gj

Sources Consulted

American Cancer Society. *Prostate Cancer National Blueprint for Action.* Developed at A Leadership Conference - Prostate Cancer in the African-American Community: An Agenda for Action, in Houston, Texas, November 20-22, 1997.

American Foundation for Urologic Disease. *Prostate Cancer - What Every Man Over 40 Should Know.* Health Reference Center, July, 1993. On-line.

Anderson, M. D. Cancer Center. *Prostate Diagnostic Center.* Orlando: Affiliated with Orlando Regional Heathcare System. On-line.

Bahn, Duke K. *Early Detection.* Rochester: Prostate Center, Crittenton Hospital in Rochester, 1997. On-line.

Bahn, Duke K. *Brachytherapy in the Treatment of Prostate Cancer: Radioactive Seed Implantation.* Rochester: Prostate Center, Crittenton Hospital in Rochester, 1997. On-line.

Balch, James F. and Phyllis A. Balch. *Prescription for Nutritional Healing.* New York: Avery Publishing Group, 1997.

Cancer Information Services. *PDQ Capsule Summary Statement.* 1997. Photocopied.

Cancer Information Services. *Cancer Facts & Figures for African Americans.* 1996. Photocopied.

Cancer Information Services. *Cancer Rates and Risks.* 1996. Photocopied.

Clinical Reference Systems. *Prostate Cancer - Care and Treatment.* Health Reference Center. December, 1994, On-line.

Clinical Reference Systems. *Prostate Cancer - Metastatis.* Health Reference Center. December, 1994. On-line.

Hendricks, Bill. *Hard Choices.* The Atlanta Journal/The Atlanta Constitution. Sunday, September 7, 1997.

Kelly, Deborah. *Survivor: 'I feel very, very lucky' to be alive.* Richmond Times-Dispatch. Thursday, June 4, 1998.

Kim, Harold E. *Radiation Therapy.* Rochester: Prostate Center, Crittenton Hospital in Rochester, 1996. On-line.

Krames Communications. *Understanding Erectile Dysfunction (Impotence): A Common and Treatable Problem.* San Bruno: 1996.

Levine, Laurence A. *Success in Treating Erectile Dysfunction: A Case Studies Monograph for the Primary Care Physician.* Rush-Presbyterian-St. Luke's Medical Center, 1998.

Mayo Clinic: Family Health Book. *Disorders of the Prostate Gland.* IVI Publishing Inc. 1993.

Mosby's Medical, Nursing, and Allied Health Dictionary. Health Reference Center. On-line.

Moul, Judd W. *Hormonal Therapy for Prostate Cancer.* US TOO International, Inc. 930 North York Road, Suite 50, Hinsdale, IL

National Cancer Institute. *Spread the Word about Cancer: A Guide for Black Americans.* NIH Publication No. 96-3412. Revised November 1995.

National Cancer Institute. *What You Need To Know About Prostate Cancer.* U.S. Department of Health and Human Service.

National Institute on Aging. *Prostate Problems.* Med Access Age Page, 1994. On-line.

National Prostate Cancer Coalition 1998 Action Plan.

Poussaint, Alvin F. "Prostate Cancer: Male Killer hits famous and not-so-famous." *Ebony.* LII, No. 6 (April 1997): 116-120, 134.

School of Medicine of the University of North Carolina at Chapel Hill. *Treating Erectile Dysfunction: New Perspectives for the Primary Care Physician.* School of Medicine of the University of North Carolina at Chapel Hill, 1998.

TAP Pharmaceuticals, Inc. *Your Health and Your Prostate.* Deerfield, Illinois. TAP Pharmaceuticals Inc., 1995.

Theragenics Corporation. *Progressive Thinking + Healing Technology (Prostate Cancer Therapy).* Norcross, GA: Theragenics Corporation.

Zeneca Pharmaceuticals. *Prostate Cancer: What it is and how it is treated.* Wilmington, Delaware. Zeneca Inc., 1996.

Celebrity
Prostate Cancer Survivors

* *Entertainer, Jerry Lewis*
* *Philanthropist, Michael Milken*
* *Singer/Entertainer, Harry Belafonte*
* *Baseball Hall-of-Famer, Stan Musial*
* *Actor, Sidney Poiter*
* *Retired General, Norman Schwarzkopf*
* *Mayor of Washington, D.C., Marion Barry*
* *New York Yankees General Manager Bob Watson*
* *Buffalo Bills, Head Coach Marv Levy*
* *Entertainer, Robert Goulet*
* *Former Archbishop Desmond Tutu*
* *Senator, Bob Dole*
* *Former Civil Rights Activist Stokely Carmichael*

Thomas L. Walker was called to pastor the Ebenezer Missionary Baptist Church in Rocky Mount, NC in 1970. At 22, he and his wife, Joyce, along with their two children, Timothy and Teresa, began a ministry that would set the standard and revolutionize the City of Rocky Mount.

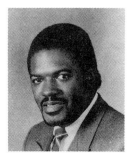

As a pastor, he has labored the past 28 years to build a ministry of excellence. TV and radio ministries, a day care center, and ministerial training are just a few of the church's outreach programs. In addition, the church has a non-profit corporation called The EBC "ATOM" Project, Inc., a program aimed at improving the quality of life for lower and middle income citizens. These initiatives are responsible for establishing Ebenzer as a paradigm for excellence.

As a community leader, he is known as one who is concerned about the common man. He served three consecutive terms as Edgecombe County Commissioner and several years as Field Representative for Congresswoman Eva M. Clayton. His leadership resulted in many positive changes in Edgecombe County, the City of Rocky Mount, the state of North Carolina, and the nation.

As a gospel recording artist, he has had his share of successes. His anointed messages of the gospel have caused many to cry "What must I do to be saved?" while his hit recording "One Day At A Time" continues to inspire the hearts of many across the nation. While writing this book, he also completed a recording project with his son, Timothy J. Walker, called "Father and Son."

Rev. Walker has always been a servant who has committed his life to improving the quality of life for others. Launching a campaign to inform men of the impending danger of prostate problems comes as no surprise to those who know him.